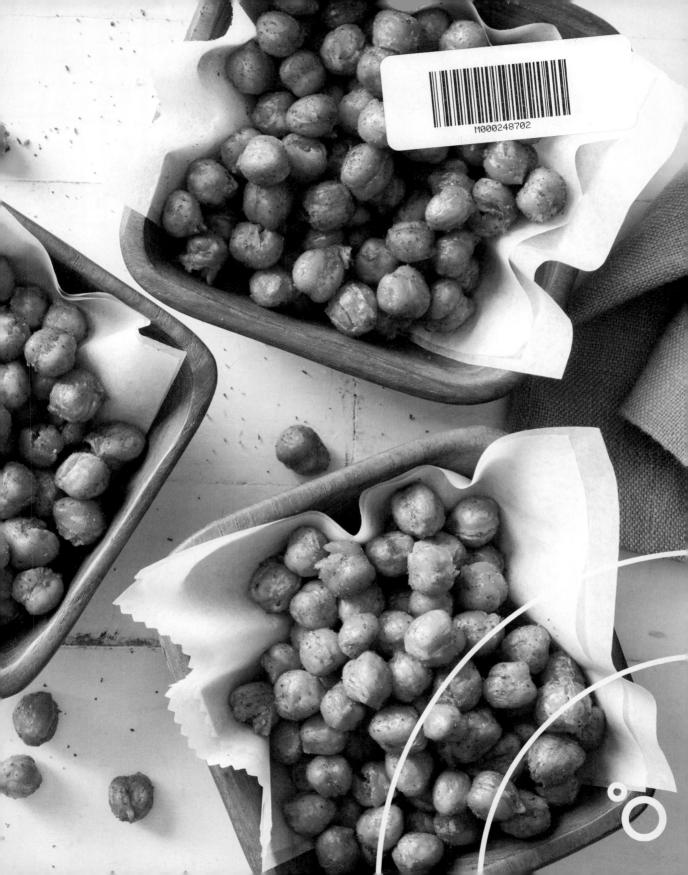

THE
NOOM
KITCHEN

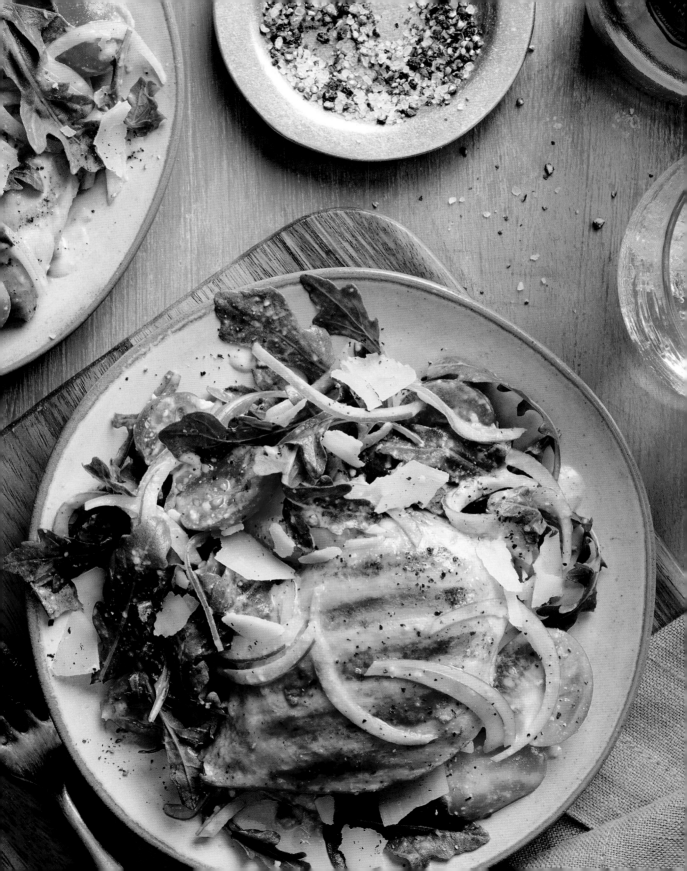

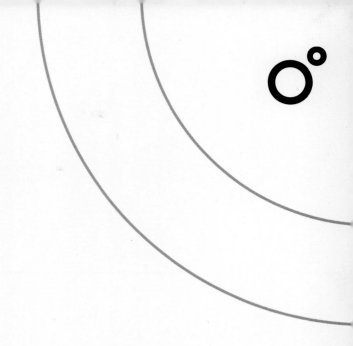

THE
NOOM
KITCHEN

◆ *100 Healthy, Delicious, Flexible Recipes for Every Day*

Recipes Developed by Adeena Sussman

SIMON ELEMENT   New York   London   Toronto   Sydney   New Delhi

SIMON ELEMENT

An Imprint of Simon & Schuster, Inc.

1230 Avenue of the Americas

New York, NY 10020

First Simon Element hardcover edition January 2024

SIMON ELEMENT is a trademark of Simon & Schuster, Inc.

Simon & Schuster: Celebrating 100 Years of Publishing in 2024

For information about special discounts for bulk purchases, please contact Simon & Schuster Special Sales at 1-866-506-1949 or business@simonandschuster.com.

The Simon & Schuster Speakers Bureau can bring authors to your live event. For more information or to book an event, contact the Simon & Schuster Speakers Bureau at 1-866-248-3049 or visit our website at www.simonspeakers.com.

Interior design by Ken Carlson, Waterbury Publications, Des Moines, IA

Manufactured in China

10 9 8 7 6 5 4 3 2 1

Library of Congress Cataloging-in-Publication Data has been applied for.

ISBN 978-1-9821-9434-5

ISBN 978-1-9821-9435-2 (ebook)

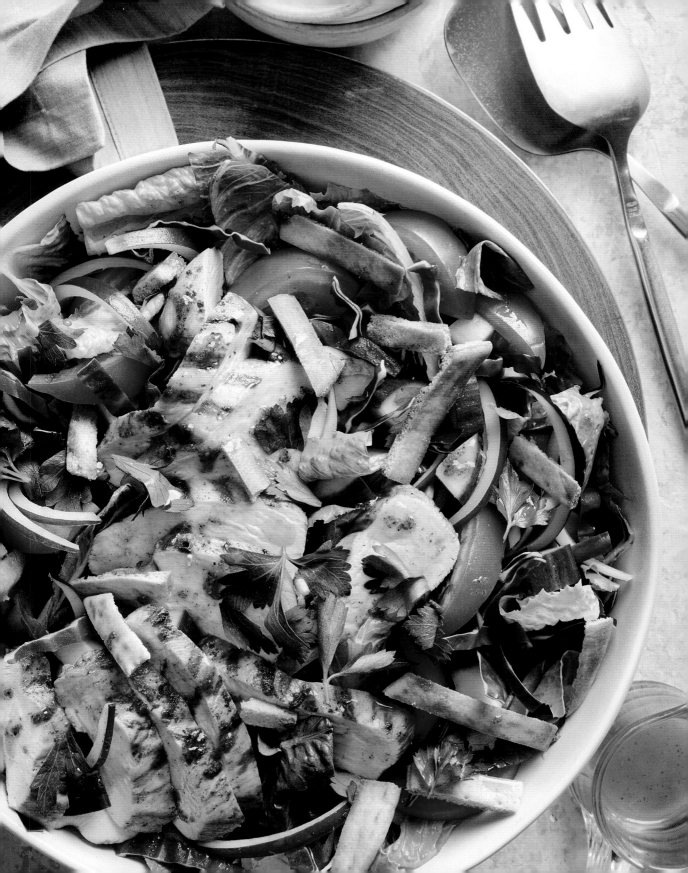

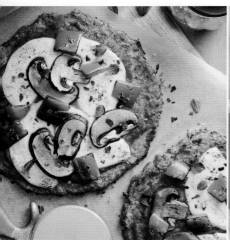
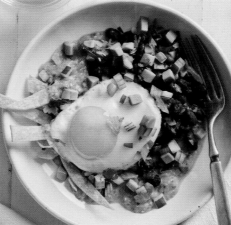
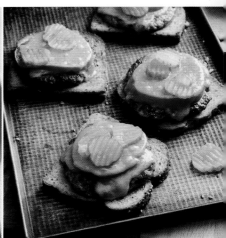

Contents

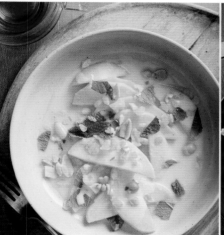
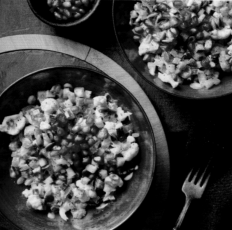
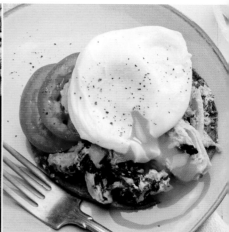

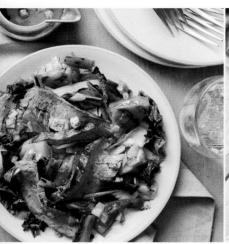
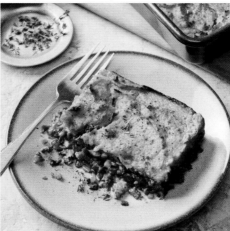
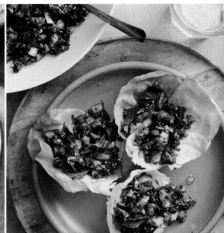

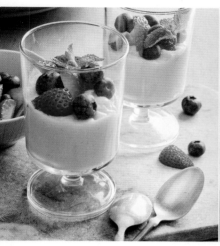
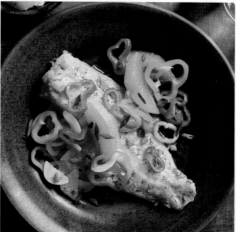
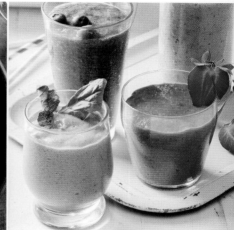

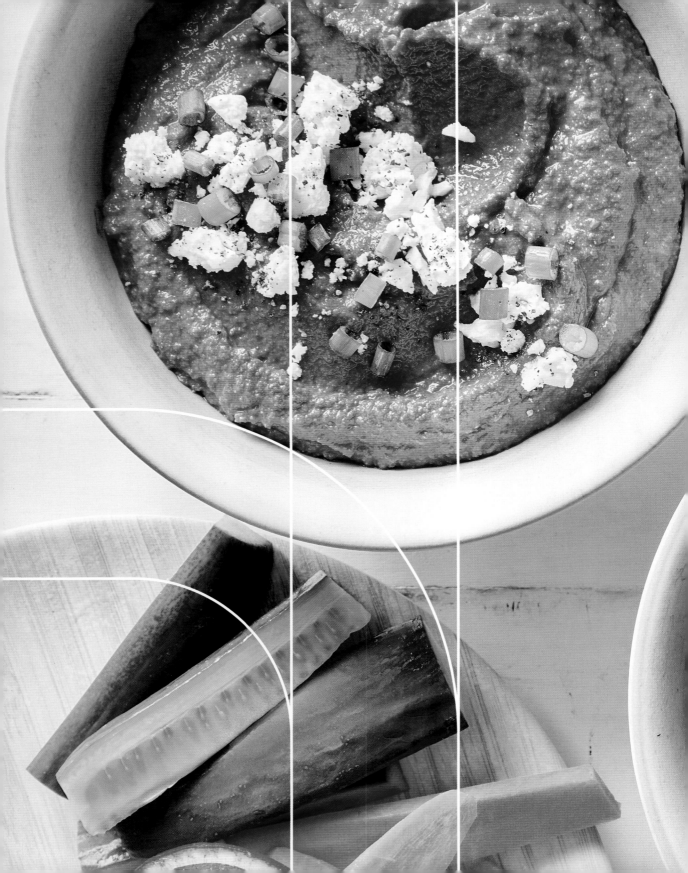

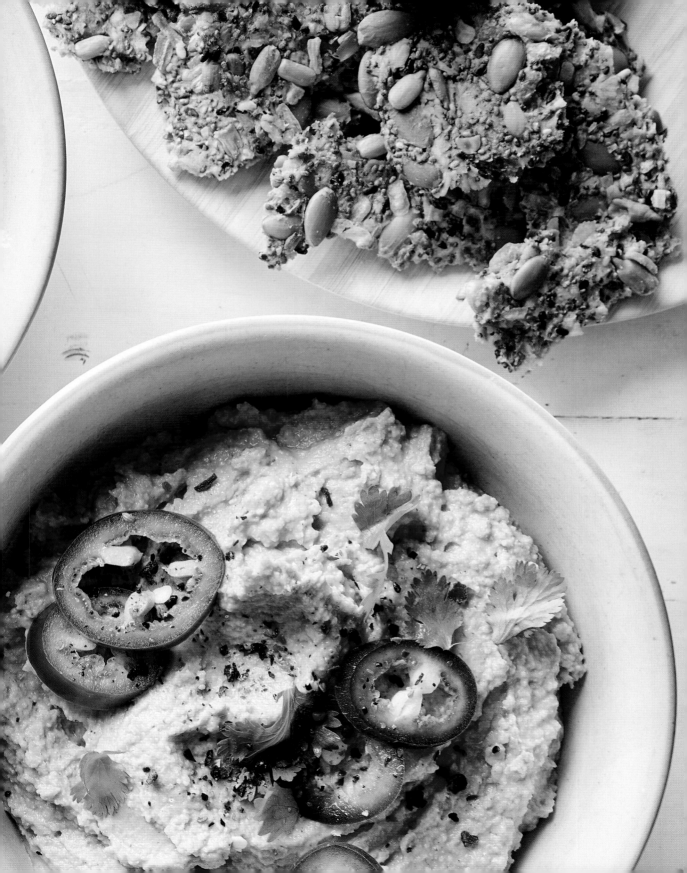

Welcome to Noom's First-Ever Cookbook

If you're looking for some creative ideas for cooking healthy but delectable meals that won't blow your calorie budget or make you feel deprived, get ready to fall in love. If you've been using the simple meal and snack ideas and the recipes on our digital platform, you're in for a treat. We're big fans of meals and snacks that take little to no prep, and we are super fans of a really great recipe. In this book, you're about to meet about 100 of those—amazing, delicious,

inventive recipes that can make your meals truly exciting, inspiring, and Noom-a-licious.

When we decided to create our very first cookbook, we had two priorities: we wanted meals that you would be excited to cook at home, and we wanted to give you lots of new ideas for eating in a way that supports your health and weight goals. We also wanted to make this cookbook easy to use, so we color-coded every recipe for you and added each one to the app meal tracker. No more hunting for similar recipes or adding every single ingredient of your favorite recipe into the app. We've got your back.

On top of all that goodness, you're going to be amazed at how many of these recipes are *green* (in the Noom-iverse, that means they have low calorie density). Many other recipes in this cookbook are *yellow* (moderately calorie dense) and a few are *orange* (calorie dense, but still nutritious). Green foods are awesome, and so are yellow and orange foods; a healthy and varied diet includes some foods from all these categories. If you've already learned how to balance your colors and eat the Noom way, you can jump right in. If not, know that reducing calorie density is part of the highly successful

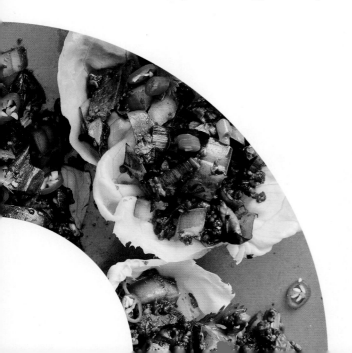

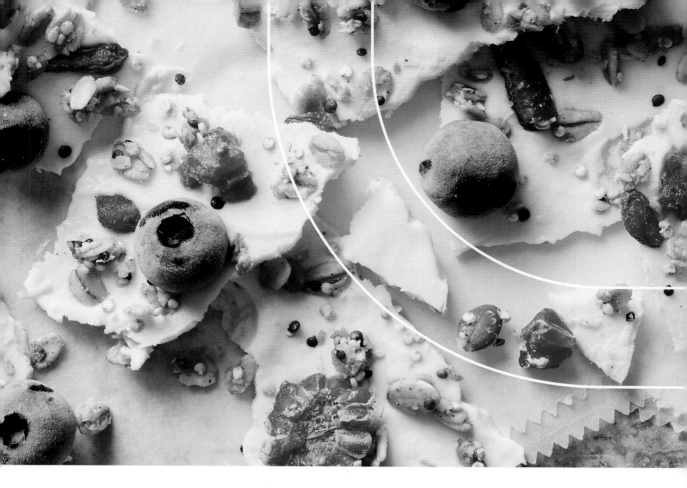

Noom formula for getting more nutrients and fewer calories out of every bite, without sacrificing taste or enjoyment.

In fact, that's the basis for the recipes in this book. We've created delicious and interesting ways to include more nutrient-dense ingredients on your plate, like fresh veggies, whole grains, protein-rich legumes, leaner chicken and beef, and seafood. Even if you're watching your portion sizes, your meals will have so much flavor that you'll feel satisfied—because what you ate was *awesome*.

Before we get into all the surprising and spectacular things you can learn to make with good old-fashioned real food, let's review some basics about our food philosophy, as well as the content of *The Noom Mindset*. Maybe this is new information for you, but if not, consider it a refresher course.

NOOM 101

First off, let's get one thing straight: Noom is not about rules and restrictions. We care about what works for you, and while we have a lot of ideas, we put them out there for you to pick and choose, according to what makes sense for your lifestyle and preferences. You don't *have* to, for instance, write down everything you eat, but if you want to try it, we are here to cheer you on and help you. We're about a lot of things at Noom: self-

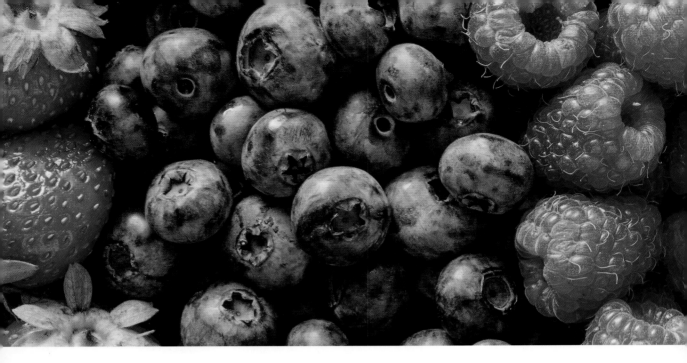

efficacy (knowing you have the power to make things happen), goal setting, habit formation, the psychology of motivation, and understanding and banishing thought distortions—those pesky untrue thoughts that creep into your head to whisper ridiculous things like "You'll never reach your goals." Ahem. *Wrong*, thought distortions. You are not welcome here!

But right now, what's on our minds is how you can feel better by upping your food game. Here are some Noom tips and psych tricks and fun facts about food and eating to help you make that happen:

There is no such thing as good or bad foods.
All foods are welcome. The more you know about the caloric and nutrient density of a food, the more you can make informed decisions about how to best meet your health goals. In this book you will find recipes for dessert, pizza, and other favorite comfort foods that we've prepared with a Noomy spin. Balance is the key, not food-shaming or guilt, and balance looks like eating

nutritious foods most of the time, and enjoying fun foods when you really want them.

Calorie density is how densely packed calories are by weight. Calorie density is a measure of how much energy is in a food by weight. For example, a grape and a raisin have the same number of calories, but because the raisin is smaller and the water has been taken out of it, it weighs less. The raisin has more calories for its weight than the grape, so the raisin is more calorie dense. That is, 1 cup of raisins has a lot more calories than 1 cup of grapes. (Helpful hint: The more water a food contains, the lower its calorie density, since water adds weight without adding calories, making the food more filling.)

Calorie-dense foods aren't bad. They are simply less filling. No moral judgment, just facts. It's fine to eat some calorie-dense foods, such as almonds or avocado. But if the majority of your diet consists of delicious foods with low calorie density, such as apples and asparagus, you will take in less energy (calories) to feel satisfied.

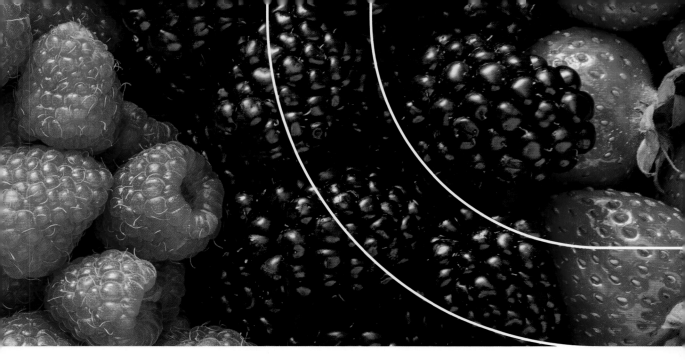

Because foods that aren't calorie dense are often nutrient dense (hello, tasty veggies), you may also get more nutrition than you were getting with a more calorically dense diet.

Nutritional density is how densely packed nutrients are by weight. Nutrient density is a lot like caloric density, but now we're looking at things like vitamins and minerals rather than energy: nutrient-dense foods have more vitamins and minerals by weight than foods that are not nutrient dense. Consider this nutrient showdown: kale versus iceberg lettuce. Kale has a lot more nutrients than iceberg lettuce, so 1 ounce of kale is more nutrient dense than 1 ounce of iceberg lettuce.

And just like calorie-dense foods aren't bad, nutrient-dense foods aren't necessarily better. Sometimes you might prefer iceberg lettuce to kale, so have what you like! Iceberg lettuce and other foods with lower nutrient density are perfectly fine choices; just remember that nutrient-dense foods deliver nutrition most

efficiently—you get more vitamins and minerals in each bite. This is all information to factor in when making your food choices.

Water and fiber are filling. Eating foods with a high water content (like those grapes versus those raisins) is one way to fill up faster. Studies show that drinking water before meals is a nice way to feel full on less food, and that can even lead to weight loss.[1] A hydrated body works better, so it's a win-win. Studies also show that fiber intake can help with weight loss,[2] if that is your goal. Fiber is also filling with few calories, and on top of that, it's great for the health of your digestion and your microbiome, so it can help keep your gut in good working order.[3]

Moderation is more sustainable than restriction. For most people, eating a balanced diet with lots of nutritious foods, plus some fun foods thrown in for pleasure, is a way to eat that is sustainable over the long term. Restricting portion sizes or certain foods may work for weight loss or other goals in the short term, but that is harder to sustain over time. Sometimes, you're really going to want that scoop of ice cream or that cheeseburger, and we at Noom want you to have them! That's all part of the joy in life. Why sit there pining away every time your friends order dessert? You can still make progress toward your goals if you enjoy fun foods once in a while. It's what you do most of the time that counts, and therein lies the secret to moderation. (And by the way, this cookbook has a lot of yummy desserts that are actually *not* calorically dense—best of both worlds!)

No matter what your dietary philosophy, you can eat well. Maybe you're low-carb or plant-based, or you eat a Mediterranean diet. Whatever philosophy you follow, as long as it doesn't drastically restrict anything, you can make healthy choices and thrive, especially if you limit (we didn't say eliminate!) processed and refined foods high in sugar, fat, and salt with little to no fiber or nutritional value.

Eating at home is a super strategy. When *you* make your meals, rather than someone on the other side of the food delivery chain or in a restaurant kitchen, you control what goes into the dish—and into *you*. You can choose to use more vegetables, less oil, more lean protein, less sugar, or whatever else you want. You can make your meals nutritious, and you can mindfully cook as well as mindfully eat. You will be participating in the creation of your own meals, so you may find that you become more invested in that and more appreciative of the process.

So, what will you make first? Maybe you'll choose to make a fabulous steak salad (page 120) or discover your new favorite way to eat bananas (page 260). Maybe you'll start the day with a black bean burrito that's so good you'll batch-cook enough for breakfast that you'll have for the whole week (page 43). Maybe you'll pair an old-fashioned roast chicken (page 137) with from-scratch French fries (page 222) and then enjoy the leftovers with our decadent brownies (page 256)! We wanted to give you recipes that show you how you can make your old favorites leaner and greener, and also inspire you to try cooking brand-new dishes with flavors you've never tried before. When you cook for yourself, you're in charge.

Besides all that, cooking is fun (seriously!), so let's get prepped.

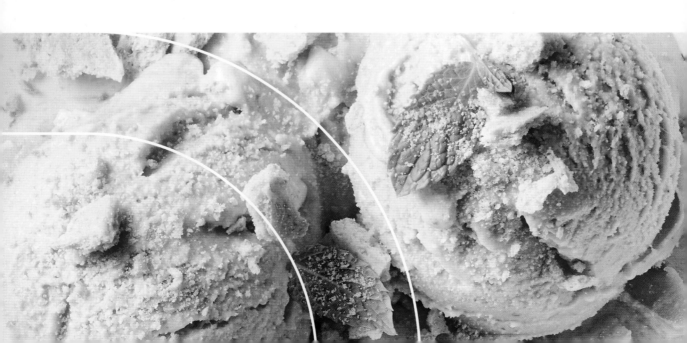

Important Things to Know About Cooking the Noom Way

The Noom Kitchen is a flavor-forward, health-conscious celebration of tastes from all around the world. The recipes in this book are for cooks of any skill level, and each is designed with Noom concepts in mind. For instance, these recipes are engineered so that orange (calorie-dense) recipes like our scrumptious Crispy Quinoa Granola (page 49) come in smaller portions. Green recipes (those with low calorie density) like Hearty Turkey Bolognese (page 123) will fill you up and keep you satisfied. Yellow recipes (those with moderate calorie density) like Spiced Chicken & Lentil Soup (page 81) are moderately portioned. We've done the balancing act for you, so go ahead—cook up a storm!

The world is full of amazing flavors that can intensify taste without compromising your health goals. The recipes in this book are inspired by many different cuisines—Mediterranean, Latin, Asian, and more. Some of these recipes may sound familiar to you, and others may be new. Some of these recipes you can probably make with ingredients you already have in your pantry; others might lead to a trip to a new part of the spice aisle. We hope you'll be excited to learn more about cooking and trying new ingredients because there is so much deliciousness in the world!

These recipes are also adaptable. If you are an improviser, use our recipes as a base and add or adjust according to your preferences. We won't take it personally! We're just happy to have you cooking with us, and we welcome and appreciate your creativity. If you're new to cooking, we think you're going to feel more and more at home in your own kitchen, the more you use this cookbook.

Here are some things to know before you get started:

Every recipe includes a color code (green, yellow, orange) at the top and nutritional information at the bottom, in case you're keeping track. For those using the app, you can enter the recipe by name into the meal tracker and a serving of the recipe you're making will automatically be entered.

Each recipe tells you how much preparation time is involved, divided into active time (meaning the time during which you'll be actively doing something, like chopping or mixing) and total time (which adds in non-active time, such as when the dish is baking in the oven). The time it takes you may not always be what's indicated (because everyone has their own style and pace of cooking), and different kitchen appliances, different combinations of ingredients, and even different climates can all affect cooking times. The times given in the recipes reflect how long it took our recipe testers to prepare each one, but your results may vary.

Nutritional analyses for each recipe do not include optional ingredients (for example, a recipe may say you can optionally add avocado or feta cheese). If there were multiple choices for a recipe ingredient, the nutritional analysis was calculated using the first choice. Also note that serving sizes are as close to accurate as possible, but your results may vary. When a recipe includes water or cooking spray, those items are not generally listed in the ingredients.

However, if the recipe asks for a particular amount of water (such as 3 tablespoons) or a specific type of cooking spray (such as olive oil cooking spray), these are listed with the ingredients.

When a recipe says "chicken breast," that means half of a full chicken breast. Most packaged chicken comes with the breasts already separated.

You can make substitutions successfully as long as the ingredients are similar. For example, you could swap green beans for asparagus, Brussels sprouts for broccoli, apples for peaches, blueberries for strawberries, chicken for turkey, lamb for beef, and so on.

Many of these recipes can be made vegetarian or vegan by substituting tofu, tempeh, or beans (like lentils or white beans) for meat. You can also substitute plant-based dairy products like almond milk or coconut yogurt for regular dairy products. Sometimes we'll give suggestions for how to do this in the recipe headnotes.

Many of these recipes can be made gluten free simply by substituting gluten-free products, such as gluten-free bread, for products made from wheat, rye, spelt, or barley.

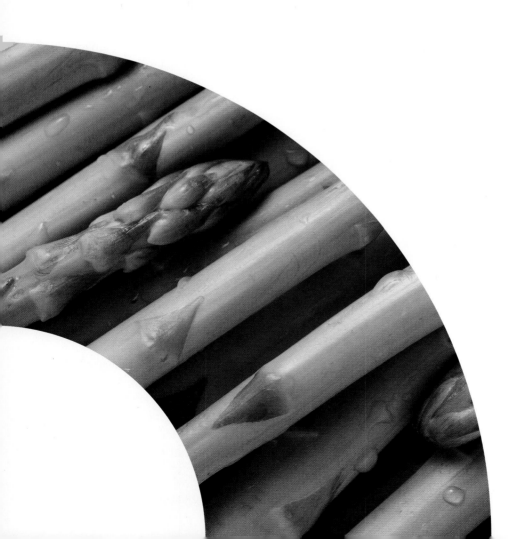

YOUR NOOM CHEF EQUIPMENT LIST

We're not going to ask you to use a lot of fancy or hard-to-find equipment. If we do mention a tool or appliance that isn't pretty common, we'll give you options for how to proceed without it. We do assume that most Noomers using this cookbook will have the following equipment on hand:

Pots and Pans

- A large nonstick skillet or sauté pan (12 inches). Good nonstick pots and pans can greatly reduce the need for oil. Just be careful to preserve the nonstick coating by using safe utensils like those made from rubber, silicone, plastic, and wood (not metal), and replace the pan when the surface becomes scratched or wears away.
- A medium nonstick skillet or sauté pan (9 to 10 inches) can also be useful for smaller amounts.
- Soup pots (or Dutch ovens) and saucepans: one large (about 6 quarts), one medium (about 4 quarts), and one small (2 or 3 quarts). These don't necessarily need to be nonstick because they're usually used for liquids.
- One or two rimmed baking sheets
- An 8- or 9-inch square baking pan and/or a 2½- to 3-quart casserole
- One or two mini muffin tins with 12 compartments

Tools

- Chef's knife or Santoku knife, which can do most chopping jobs—keep it sharp for safety, and watch your fingers
- Paring knife, for peeling veggies and small chopping jobs like mincing garlic
- Cutting board (plastic, bamboo, wood)
- Spatula, for flipping
- Rubber scraper, to get every last drop out of pans and bowls
- Stirring spoons (wooden or plastic, to protect your nonstick pans)
- Slotted spoon, for poached eggs and stubby pasta

- Measuring cups: 1 cup, ½ cup, ⅓ cup, ¼ cup
- Measuring spoons: 1 tablespoon, 1 teaspoon, ½ teaspoon, ¼ teaspoon
- Colander, for draining pasta and rinsing vegetables and fruits
- Fine-mesh strainer, for draining things that will fall through the larger holes of a colander (rice, quinoa, etc.)
- Can opener
- Cheese grater, which is good for grating vegetables, too
- Wooden or metal skewers, for grilling or making kabobs
- Oven mitts or pot holders...because pans get hot
- Meat thermometer, to make sure your dinner isn't still raw in the middle, or overcooked— instant-read thermometers are quick and handy
- Sealable plastic bags, for a million reasons
- Sealable containers of various sizes, for marinating and storage
- Clean kitchen towels

Small appliances

- Blender, for smoothies, sauces, and pureed soups
- Electric hand-held mixer, for mixing batter

Optional but nice to have:

- Food processor, for faster, easier chopping
- Food scale, for getting really precise about amounts and portion sizes, if that's your thing
- Immersion blender, to puree soups right in the pot
- Mandoline, for easy, even slicing
- Microplane, for grating things really finely, like citrus peel or Parmesan cheese
- Pressure cooker, for cooking things faster, especially dried beans
- Slow cooker, for cooking things slower, like all-day soups, stews, stock, or roasts
- Small plates—they make small portions seem more satisfying. Many Noomers swear by this strategy.
- Stand mixer, for heavy-duty mixing jobs and kneading bread (really only useful if you bake a lot)

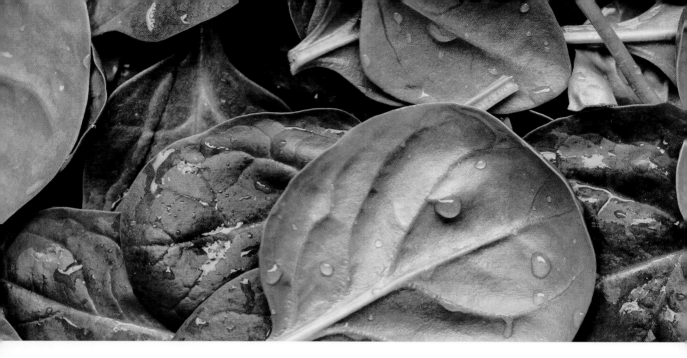

YOUR NOOMY PANTRY, FRIDGE, AND FREEZER

This book's recipes call for many basic, easy-to-find ingredients and a few specialty ingredients, many of those optional. We expect you'll shop for specific ingredients as you need them, but this is a list of pretty much everything you'll need to make the recipes in this book.

Seasonal Fruits and Veggies

Seasonal fruits and veggies are fresher, tastier, juicier, and quite possibly more nutritious—especially if they are locally produced, since nutrient content is highest right after harvest. (They also tend to be less expensive.) To boost the nutrient density of your menu, try choosing your produce according to the season. Here's a quick start guide:

Winter

- Beets
- Brussels sprouts
- Grapefruit
- Kiwi fruit
- Leeks
- Lemons
- Oranges
- Potatoes
- Sweet potatoes
- Winter squash

Spring

- Apricots
- Asparagus
- Baby lettuces and baby spinach
- Broccoli
- Carrots
- Mushrooms
- Peas
- Radishes
- Rhubarb
- Strawberries
- Swiss chard

Summer

- Avocados
- Bell peppers
- Blueberries
- Cantaloupe
- Cherries
- Eggplant
- Peaches
- Plums
- Raspberries
- Summer squash
- Tomatoes
- Watermelon

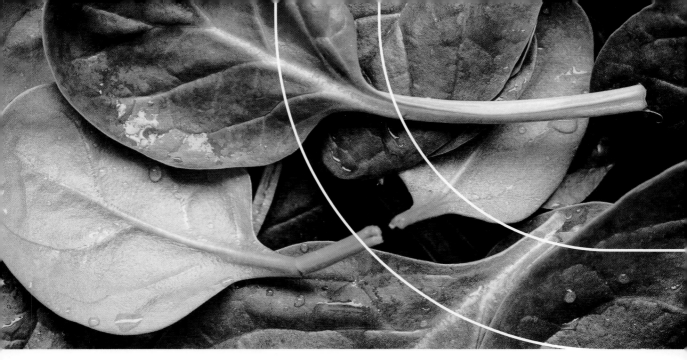

Fall

- Apples
- Cauliflower
- Cranberries
- Grapes
- Kale
- Parsnips
- Pears
- Pumpkin
- Rutabagas
- Turnips

Vegetables (fresh and frozen as available)

Veggies are the cornerstone of a nutrient-dense, non-calorically-dense diet. We recommend loading up at every opportunity! And don't worry about a produce bin full of veggies gone bad—frozen fruits and veggies are a perfectly nutritious alternative. If you bought too much of something, just rinse it, dry it, and freeze it for later.

- Avocado
- Beets (vacuum-packed cooked beets are convenient)
- Bell peppers (green, yellow, orange, red)
- Butternut squash
- Cabbage
- Carrots
- Cauliflower
- Celery
- Dried shiitake mushrooms (and other types if you want to experiment)
- Garlic
- Green beans
- Jalapeño
- Leafy greens: We like to keep a variety of mixed lettuces, spring mix, spinach, arugula, chard, kale, collard greens, etc., on hand. One of the best ways to reduce the caloric density of your recipes is to add a handful of greens. If you ate a big salad every day, we would be impressed. #Goals
- Leeks
- Mushrooms (button and portobello)
- Onions (yellow, white, red)
- Persian cucumbers (these mini cukes have a thinner, more tender skin)
- Scallions
- Shallots
- Tomatoes
- Zucchini

Fruit (fresh and frozen as available)

Basic year-round fruit is great for snacking. If you always have apples, bananas, blueberries, and oranges available to grab and go, you're already ahead of the game. Keep some fruit in the freezer too, for smoothies.

- Apples
- Bananas
- Blueberries
- Figs (fresh or dried)
- Lemons
- Limes
- Mangoes
- Oranges
- Pineapple
- Pomegranate seeds (also called arils)
- Strawberries

Whole Grains

Whole grains have more fiber and are more filling and nutrient dense than refined grains. Some of our faves to keep around at all times:

- Brown rice
- Corn tortillas
- Flours: We like to keep both whole-grain and white whole wheat or whole wheat pastry flour on hand. If you are gluten free, you could substitute brown rice or cassava flour, or another gluten-free flour, for thickening. For baking, you will need a tried-and-true gluten-free baking mix if you can't use wheat flour.
- Oatmeal (and oat milk)
- Quinoa
- Shirataki noodles (made from a vegetable root, so not technically a grain)
- Whole wheat bread, tortillas, pita bread, sandwich thins
- Whole-grain pastas, including spaghetti, penne, couscous, and orzo, and pastas made from spelt, brown rice, etc.

Legumes (dried or canned)

Fiber rich, nutrient dense, protein packed, and virtually fat free, legumes are super foods in our (literal) book. Dried legumes are economical, but you need to soak them overnight before cooking (or use a pressure cooker). Canned legumes cost a bit more but are still pretty inexpensive and convenient. Some types to keep on hand:

- Black beans
- Cannellini beans
- Chickpeas (garbanzo beans)
- Edamame (fresh or frozen)
- Kidney beans
- Lentils (brown or green and beluga or French)
- Pinto beans
- White beans

Oils

A lot of the recipes in this book use a little bit of oil for flavor and to grease pans. You don't need much oil to make sure your food doesn't stick and to make a recipe taste decadent:

- Coconut oil
- Cooking spray
- Extra-virgin olive oil
- Grapeseed oil, for when you need a neutral flavor
- Olive oil cooking spray
- Peanut oil, for frying

Dairy and Eggs

Eggs are a great source of protein, and other dairy items like butter, cheese, and yogurt add a lot of flavor, even if they are sometimes more calorie dense. Again, you don't need much!

- Butter, unsalted (we use it sparingly)
- Eggs, large
- Feta or goat cheese, which pack a lot of flavor with just a sprinkling
- Milk (nonfat, low-fat, or plant-based)
- Parmigiano-Reggiano cheese, for adding a lot of flavor
- Swiss cheese, reduced-fat
- Yogurt (plain unsweetened regular or nonfat Greek)

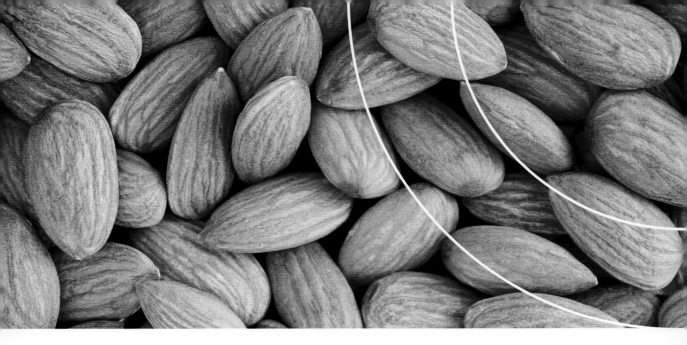

Protein foods (animal and vegetable)

Protein is what muscles are made of, so be sure to get enough, especially on workout days. Eat these within a few days of buying them, or keep them in the freezer until you need them.

- Beef, lean ground and lean cuts
- Chicken breasts
- Chicken, ground
- Deli ham
- Salmon
- Shrimp
- Tempeh (fermented soybean cake)
- Tofu (extra-firm and soft silken)
- Tuna, canned albacore
- Turkey, ground
- Turkey sausage, hot or sweet Italian style

Nuts and Seeds

A good protein source, nuts and seeds are generally orange foods, but in small amounts they can make a recipe more satisfying. They are also packed with nutrients.

- Almond butter
- Almond milk (unsweetened plain and vanilla)
- Almonds
- Chia seeds
- Coconut milk (unsweetened, the kind in a carton, not a can)
- Coconut water with no added sweetener (for smoothies and general hydration)
- Flax seeds (ground to make their nutrients more available to your system)
- Hazelnuts
- Peanut butter (natural unsweetened)
- Peanuts (technically a legume, but we think of them as nutty)
- Pecans
- Pumpkin seeds
- Sesame seeds
- Sunflower seeds
- Tahini (sesame paste)
- Walnuts

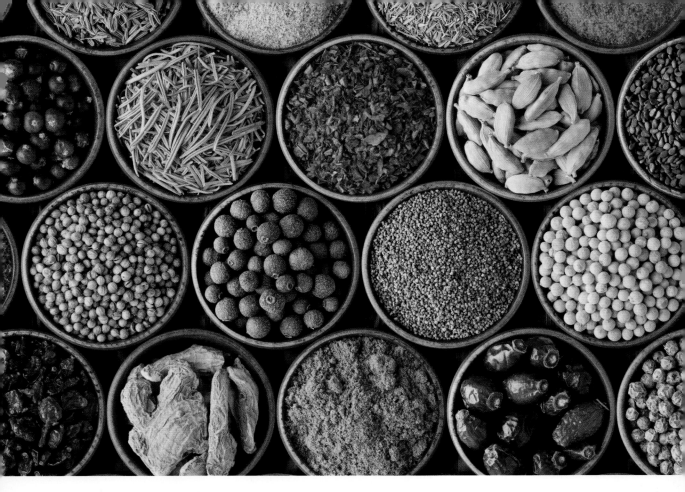

Flavor Bombs and Other Specialty Ingredients

You'll find that the recipes in this book occasionally call for ingredients that are extra loaded with flavor. In fact, many of these items are the secret ingredients in the recipes for obtaining maximum flavor with minimum calorie density.

- Apple cider vinegar
- Artichoke hearts, canned
- Black bean sauce (a fermented sauce)
- Broth: Beef, chicken, vegetable—you can sauté in broth instead of oil to reduce caloric density

- Canned tomatillos
- Red pepper flakes
- Chili oil
- Dijon mustard
- Filé powder (finely ground sassafras leaves; traditionally used as a thickener in gumbo)
- Fish sauce
- Flaky sea salt, for garnish
- Gochujang (a Korean spicy chili paste)
- Goji berries, dried
- Harissa (a Tunisian chili paste)
- Hearts of palm, canned
- Matcha powder
- Piri piri sauce, a spicy African chili sauce

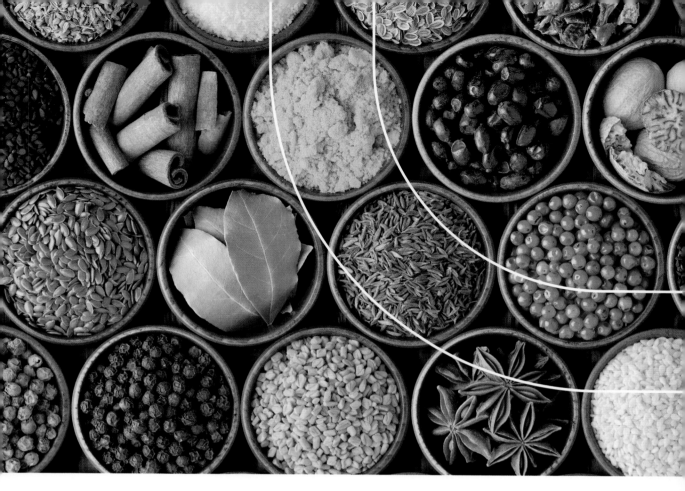

- Pomegranate molasses
- Preserved lemon
- Rice vinegar/rice wine vinegar
- Sumac powder (ground leaves, a red-colored spice popular in Middle Eastern cooking)
- Sweetened condensed milk
- Tahini (sesame paste)
- White vinegar
- Worcestershire sauce
- Za'atar (Middle Eastern spice mixture typically including sesame seeds, sumac, and salt)

Herbs and Spices (dried or fresh)

Herbs and spices are another great way to add flavor without adding fat and calories.

- Basil
- Bay leaf
- Cardamom
- Cilantro
- Cinnamon
- Cumin
- Dill
- Garlic
- Ginger
- Kosher salt
- Mint
- Nutmeg
- Oregano
- Paprika, sweet and smoked
- Parsley
- Sea salt
- Thyme
- Turmeric

Techniques

HOW TO POACH AN EGG

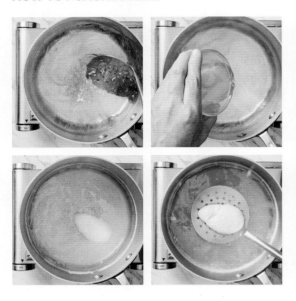

1. Line a large plate with a clean towel.

2. Crack an egg into a small bowl or ramekin. Fill a small saucepan with water. Bring to a boil over high heat, then add 1 teaspoon white vinegar, turn the heat to medium, and swirl the water. Slip the egg into the water and cook until the white is opaque, 2 to 3 minutes.

3. Remove the egg with a slotted spoon and place on a towel-lined plate.

HOW TO SECTION AN ORANGE

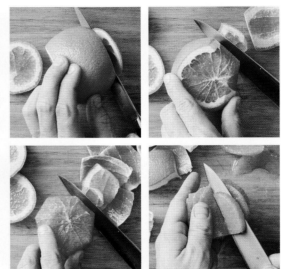

1. Use a sharp knife to cut off the top and bottom of an orange. Stand the orange on a cutting board with a rim and cut the peel and rind from the orange, following the shape of the fruit and trying to cut off as little of the flesh as possible.

2. Gently cut between the white membranes that divide the flesh of the orange wedges. Squeeze the membrane to release any juice; reserve as needed for your recipe.

3. Move the orange flesh into a bowl, discarding the remaining web of orange membranes and as many pits as you can.

HOW TO ASSEMBLE A SUSHI HAND ROLL

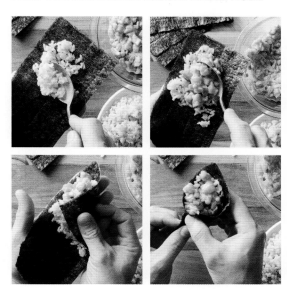

HOW TO ROLL A SUMMER ROLL

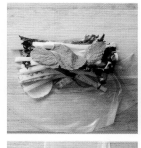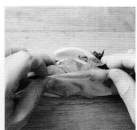

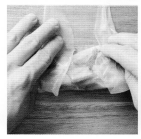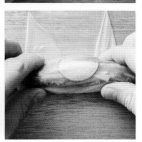

1. Fill a small bowl with water for moistening the nori.

2. Arrange a sheet of nori with the longer side parallel to the bottom of your clean work surface. Spoon 2 tablespoons of prepared rice onto the center of one side of the nori, at least ½ inch from the edge.

3. Spoon about ⅓ cup of salmon or other seafood mixture on top of the rice.

4. Pull one near corner of the nori over the filling, then continue to roll the nori into a cone shape, with the filling exposed on the top. (If some filling spills out, you can spoon in a bit more once the cone is complete.)

5. Moisten the corner of the nori on the outside of the cone and seal it to the cone.

1. Fill a clean skillet or rimmed tray with warm tap water (replenish with more warm tap water as necessary to maintain temperature). Arrange a clean, dampened towel on a clean work surface.

2. Dip 1 rice wrapper into the water; moisten it for a few seconds until it begins to soften but is not completely translucent. Remove the wrapper from the water and place it on the damp towel.

3. Arrange 1 or 2 basil leaves in the center of the wrapper, about 2½ inches from the edge. Arrange 2 or 3 radish rounds, about 4 strips of tofu, and some carrots on top.

4. Center 2 or 3 lettuce pieces on top, then top them with a strip of mango and 2 or 3 small mint leaves.

5. Roll the summer rolls: Line a large plate with a damp paper towel. Gently pull the bottom of the wrapper over the filling, then fold in the sides as though you're making a burrito. Roll up and place the roll on the plate. Cover the roll with another damp paper towel.

HOW TO ASSEMBLE BANANA LOTI

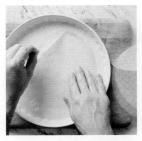
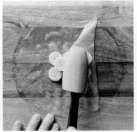
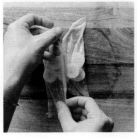
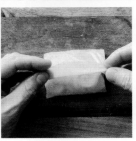

1. Arrange 6 banana slices in 3 rows of 2 slices each in the center of a rice wrapper (to form a sort of rectangle), then stack 2 more slices on top for a total of 8 slices on the wrapper.

2. Using a silicone spatula and your hands, gently fold the sides of the wrapper over the banana slices, then fold in the top and bottom to form a rectangular pocket.

HOW TO SCRAPE GRANITA

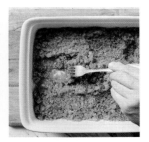

1. Remove the pan from the freezer after 30 minutes. The granita should just be starting to solidify around the edges.

2. Using a fork, scrape the icy bits from the side and return the pan to the freezer. Set a timer for 30 minutes.

3. After 30 minutes, remove the pan from the freezer and scrape the icy bits again.

4. Repeat this procedure every 30 minutes for 5 or 6 times, or between 2½ and 3 hours, so the granita never freezes solid and stays in a coarse state. Keep scraping the ice from the sides and bottom, breaking up larger chunks. The granita should be fully frozen.

HOW TO MAKE CHICKEN CUTLETS

1. Place a large, boneless chicken breast (about 8 ounces) on a cutting board.

2. Gently press down on the breast with the palm of your hand and, using a sharp knife, very carefully cut it in half horizontally to create two 4-ounce cutlets. (This is a little bit easier if the chicken isn't fully defrosted, making it firmer and easier to slice.) Watch your fingers!

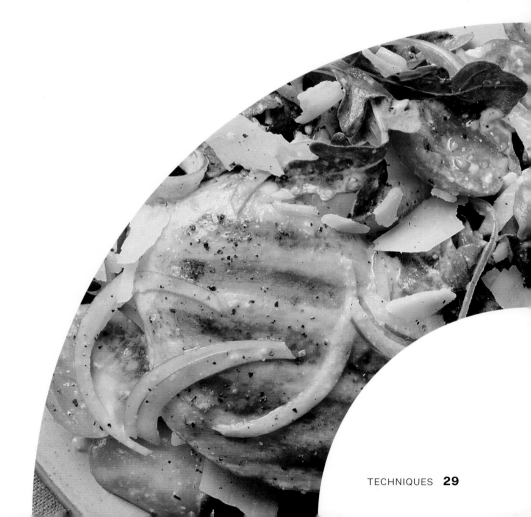

Breakfasts and Brunches

Is breakfast the most important meal of the day? We think every meal is important, but that certainly includes breakfast (or brunch, if you're in that kind of mood). Let these recipes inspire your resolve to begin your day on a high note.

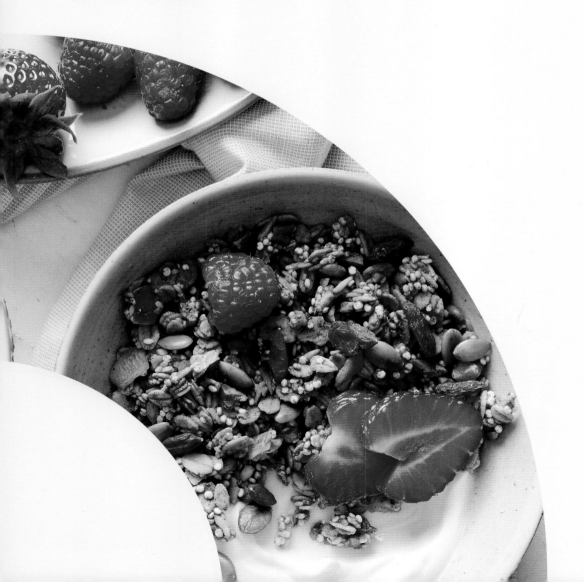

Chai-Spiced Overnight Oats

Old-fashioned rolled whole-grain oats have more fiber and protein per serving than quick oats, better nutritional density, and great flavor! If you are cooking oats, you'll find that steel-cut or Irish oats have even more nutritional density, but they aren't good for overnight oats, so save them for when you are firing up the stove or slow cooker.

You can make this entire recipe and store all six servings in your refrigerator so you have breakfast ready to go for an entire week. You are *so efficient.*

2⅓ cups unsweetened vanilla almond milk

1½ cups old-fashioned rolled oats

2 tablespoons pure maple syrup

2 tablespoons chia seeds

1 teaspoon vanilla extract

½ teaspoon ground cinnamon

½ teaspoon ground ginger

¼ teaspoon ground cardamom

¼ teaspoon sea salt

Pinch of finely ground black pepper (optional)

¾ cup fresh or defrosted frozen blueberries (or another fruit you enjoy)

¾ cup diced fresh or defrosted frozen mango (or another fruit you enjoy)

SERVES 6 **TOTAL TIME:** 4 HOURS 10 MINUTES (INCLUDING CHILLING)

1. Prepare and chill the oats: To a medium bowl, add the almond milk, oats, maple syrup, chia seeds, vanilla, cinnamon, ginger, cardamom, salt, and black pepper if using, and mix until well combined. Gently fold in ½ cup each of the blueberries and mango.

2. Divide the mixture among 6 glasses or jars, seal tightly with plastic or lids, and refrigerate at least 4 hours.

3. Finish and serve the oatmeal: Remove the glasses from the refrigerator, uncover, and top each with the remaining blueberries and mango.

Note: Overnight oats can be refrigerated, tightly sealed, in an airtight container for up to 5 days.

NUTRITIONAL INFORMATION (1 SERVING = GENEROUS ½ CUP) Calories 159, Total Fat 4.2 g 6%, Saturated Fat 0.5 g 2%, Trans Fat 0.1 g, Cholesterol 0.0 mg 0%, Sodium 150.4 mg 6%, Total Carb 28.1 g 9%, Dietary Fiber 5.3 g 21%, Sugars 10.2 g, Added Sugars 0 g, Protein 4.1 g 8%, Vitamin D 0.0 mcg 0%, Calcium 220.2 mg 22%, Iron 1.6 mg 9%, Potassium 153.3 mg 4%

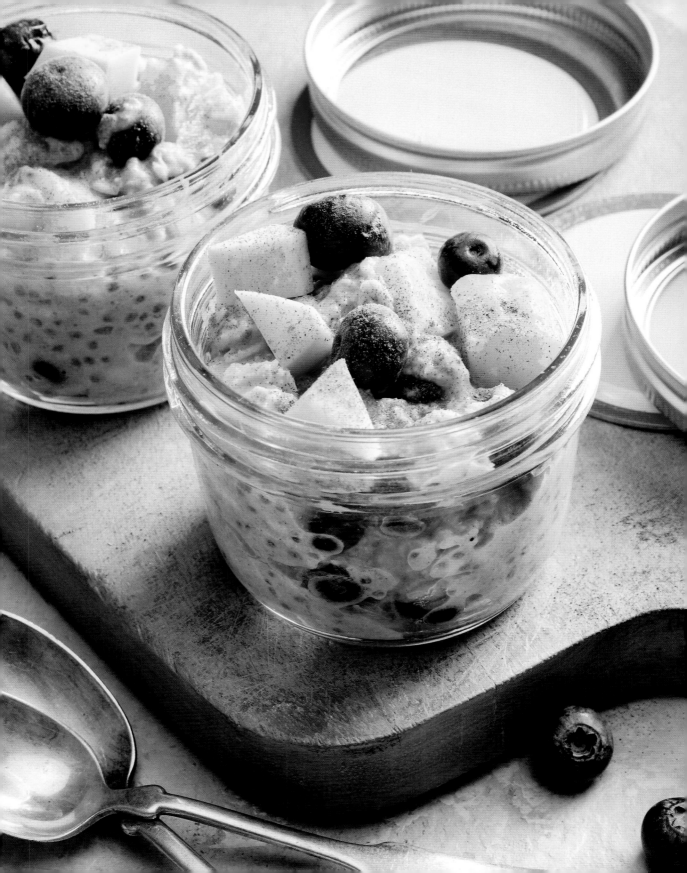

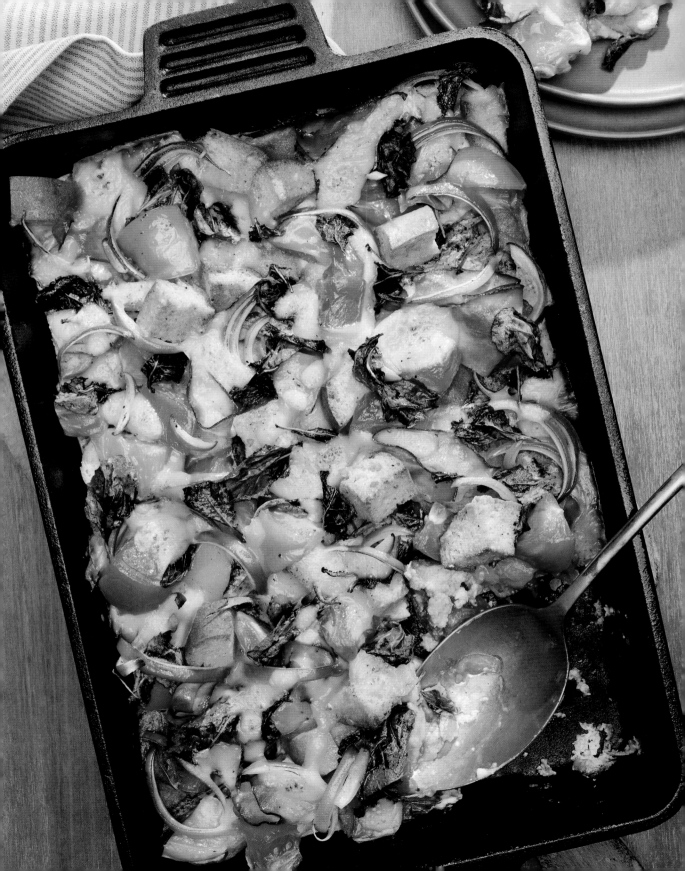

Ham & Swiss Breakfast Strata

If you're into the '80s, you might be having a flashback—that was the heyday of strata, but we think it deserves a revival because it's so simple to make and so, so good. Traditional strata is supposed to sit overnight in the refrigerator to let the egg mixture soak into the bread, and you can do that if you're at all into prepping your meals. Or you can make it when you wake up, let it sit for two hours, then bake it just in time for brunch.

8 ounces day-old whole-grain baguette (or other leftover whole-grain bread), cubed (about 5 cups)

2 large vine-ripened tomatoes, cored and cut into 1-inch cubes

2 cups fresh baby spinach or baby kale leaves

4 ounces reduced-fat Swiss cheese, shredded or cut into thin strips

4 ounces thinly sliced smoked ham

½ small red onion, thinly sliced

1½ cups nonfat milk

6 large eggs

1 tablespoon Dijon mustard

2 teaspoons kosher salt

¼ teaspoon freshly ground black pepper

SERVES 8 TOTAL TIME: 3 HOURS 25 MINUTES

1. Prepare the strata base: Spray a 9-inch square (2½-quart) baking dish with cooking spray. Arrange the bread cubes in the baking dish, then nestle in the tomatoes, spinach, cheese, ham, and onion evenly in the baking dish, letting some of the ham peek out the top.

2. Make the custard and chill the strata: In a medium bowl, whisk the milk, eggs, mustard, salt, and pepper until smooth and fully combined. Pour the liquid mixture evenly over the bread mixture, moving pieces of bread to ensure the liquid reaches the bottom of the dish. Cover and refrigerate for at least 2 hours and up to 12 hours.

3. Bake and serve the strata: Take the strata out of the refrigerator 1 hour before you plan to bake it. Preheat the oven to 350°F.

4. Bake the strata until the top is crusty but the center is not dried out, 60 to 70 minutes. Let cool for 10 minutes, then cut into 8 pieces and serve.

NUTRITIONAL INFORMATION (1 SERVING = ⅛ OF THE STRATA) Calories 206, Total Fat 6.8 g 10%, Saturated Fat 2.5 g 13%, Trans Fat 0.1 g, Cholesterol 150.5 mg 50%, Sodium 820.5 mg 34%, Total Carb 19.5 g 6%, Dietary Fiber 2.7 g 11%, Sugars 5.2 g, Added Sugars 0 g, Protein 17.3 g 35%, Vitamin D 52.5 mcg 13%, Calcium 245 mg 25%, Iron 2.4 mg 13%, Potassium 334.9 mg 10%

NOOM CHEF'S TIP: STRATA VARIATIONS *Strata is endlessly accommodating. Whatever veggies and protein you have on hand will work tucked in between the baguette cubes and flavored with eggs and a bit of cheese. Strata is a great way to use up bread that's getting a little stale, but if you want to ditch the grains altogether, substitute about 4 cups of roasted cauliflower for the bread cubes. Now that's thinking outside the (bread) box!*

Spicy Tomato & Red Pepper Shakshuka

Shakshuka is a traditional breakfast dish of eggs simmered in a spicy, savory tomato sauce. It's easy, nourishing, delicious, and nutritionally dense, but not calorically dense. Shakshuka is traditionally served with a lot of tasty toppings, such as avocado cubes, olive slices, or crumbled feta. Just remember that these extras are not counted in the nutritional analysis of this recipe.

1 tablespoon olive oil

1 small onion, sliced

1 medium red bell pepper, seeded and diced

2 large garlic cloves, thinly sliced

2 tablespoons tomato paste

¾ teaspoon ground cumin

¾ teaspoon smoked paprika

¼ teaspoon ground turmeric

2 14½-ounce cans crushed tomatoes

2 teaspoons finely chopped jalapeño (optional; seeded, if desired), plus more for serving

½ cup water

½ teaspoon kosher salt, plus more for seasoning

4 large eggs

¼ cup chopped scallion greens

SERVES 4   TOTAL TIME: 40 MINUTES

1. Prepare the sauce: Heat the olive oil in a large (12-inch) skillet over medium heat, then add the onion and bell pepper and cook, stirring, until the onion is lightly golden, 8 to 10 minutes. Add the garlic and cook, stirring often, for 1 more minute.

2. Add the tomato paste, cumin, paprika, and turmeric and cook until the mixture is fragrant and the tomato paste is slightly caramelized, about 2 minutes, stirring constantly.

3. Add the tomatoes, jalapeño if using, water, and ½ teaspoon salt. Bring to a boil, then reduce the heat to low and simmer until the sauce has darkened and thickened slightly, 10 to 15 minutes. It may bubble and spatter, so adjust the temperature as needed and stir periodically. Taste and season with additional salt if you think it needs more.

4. Assemble and bake the shakshuka: Use a spoon to form 4 wells in the sauce. Crack an egg into each well. Cover the skillet and cook the eggs until the whites are no longer runny, about 5 minutes.

5. Garnish and serve: Top the shakshuka with the scallion greens and any additional desired toppings. Serve family style.

Note: Store any leftovers, covered, in the refrigerator for up to 2 days.

NUTRITIONAL INFORMATION (1 SERVING = 1 EGG, PLUS 1 CUP SAUCE) Calories 200, Total Fat 9 g 14%, Saturated Fat 2.2 g 11%, Trans Fat 0.1 g, Cholesterol 186 mg 62%, Sodium 597.4 mg 25%, Total Carb 22.4 g 7%, Dietary Fiber 5.9 g 23%, Sugars 12.6 g, Added Sugars 0 g, Protein 10.9 g 22%, Vitamin D 41 mcg 10%, Calcium 118.7 mg 12%, Iron 4.4 mg 25%, Potassium 905.4 mg 26%

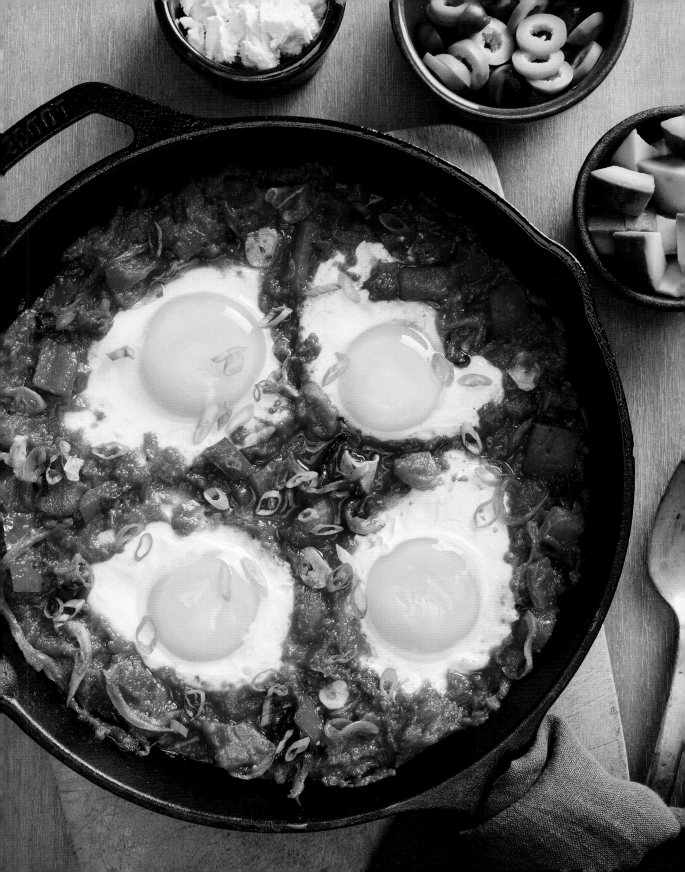

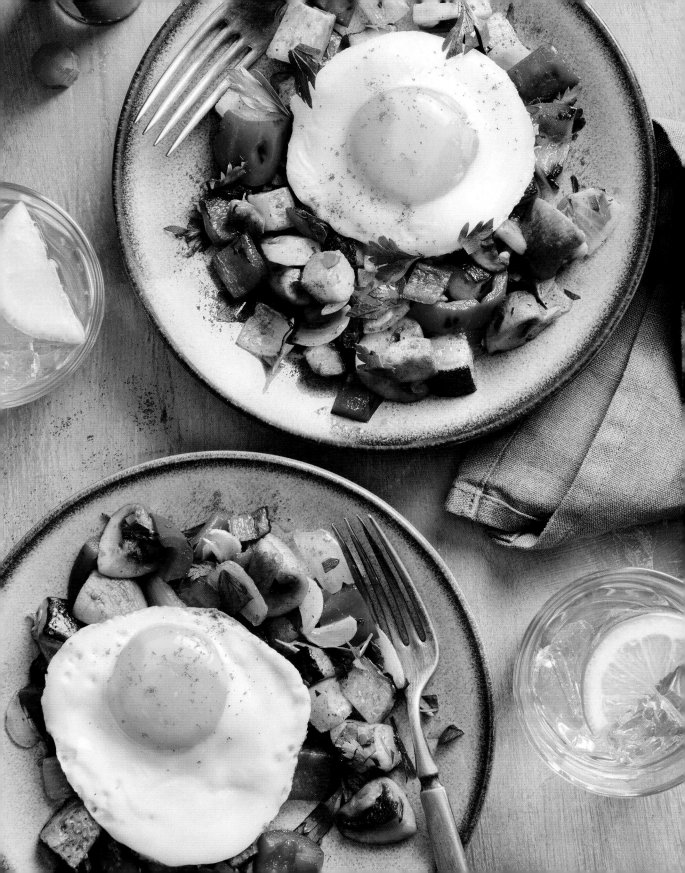

Sunny-Side-Up Hash

A good hash is yum with eggs for brunch, but it typically means a lot of starchy potatoes and oil. Not in this sleek and savory vegetarian version! This hash is all non-starchy veggies. The mushrooms and zucchini give it a meaty texture, while plenty of onions and bell peppers make it filling and nutritious. Note that if you prefer to eat plant-based, some crumbled extra-firm tofu can stand in for the eggs.

1½ tablespoons olive oil

8 ounces white button mushrooms, trimmed of stems and quartered

1 medium zucchini (about 6 ounces), cut unto ½-inch cubes

¾ teaspoon kosher salt

1 large onion, diced

1 large green bell pepper, diced

1 large red bell pepper, diced

1 small jalapeño, seeded and diced (optional)

3 garlic cloves, thinly sliced

1 teaspoon ground cumin

½ teaspoon smoked paprika

¼ cup chopped fresh parsley, plus more for garnish

4 large eggs

Hot sauce (optional; for serving)

SERVES 4 TOTAL TIME: 15 MINUTES

1. Make the hash: Heat 1 tablespoon of the olive oil in an extra-large (12- to 14-inch), heavy skillet over medium-high heat. Add the mushrooms, zucchini, and ¼ teaspoon salt and cook, stirring every 1 to 2 minutes, until the vegetables are browned and slightly dried out, 5 to 6 minutes total. Remove to a plate.

2. Add the remaining ½ tablespoon oil to the skillet, then add the onion, green and red bell peppers, jalapeño (if using), and the remaining ½ teaspoon salt. Cook, stirring occasionally, until the peppers wilt and char slightly, 6 to 7 minutes.

3. Add the garlic, cumin, and smoked paprika and cook, stirring, until fragrant, about 2 minutes.

4. Return the mushrooms and zucchini to the pan and cook, stirring, until warmed through, 1 to 2 minutes. Stir in ¼ cup parsley and cover to keep warm.

5. Cook the eggs: Spray a large (12-inch) nonstick skillet with cooking spray and heat over medium heat.

6. Crack 2 eggs into the skillet and cook until the whites are set but the yolks are still runny, 2 to 3 minutes. Carefully remove the eggs to a plate. Repeat with more cooking spray and the remaining eggs. (If your skillet is big enough, you can cook all 4 eggs at the same time.)

7. Assemble the dish and serve: Divide the hash among 4 plates and top each plate with a sunny-side-up egg. Garnish with more parsley and serve with hot sauce, if using.

NUTRITIONAL INFORMATION (1 SERVING = 1 EGG, PLUS 1 CUP HASH) Calories 179, Total Fat 10.4 g 16%, Saturated Fat 2.4 g 12%, Trans Fat 0.1 g, Cholesterol 186 mg 62%, Sodium 421.7 mg 18%, Total Carb 13.1 g 4%, Dietary Fiber 3.6 g 15%, Sugars 6.9 g, Added Sugars 0 g, Protein 10.1 g 20%, Vitamin D 45 mcg 11%, Calcium 63.1 mg 6%, Iron 2.1 mg 12%, Potassium 636.3 mg 18%

Spinach-Artichoke Dip Eggs Benedict

This breakfast looks and tastes so special, you'll feel like you're having breakfast in a fancy café. This version is healthier (and less calorically dense) than the restaurant versions because whole-grain sandwich thins stand in for English muffins, and the creamy spinach-artichoke dip (inspired!) is lightened up with nonfat Greek yogurt.

FOR THE EGGS BENEDICT

3 whole-grain sandwich thins, split in half

Spinach-Artichoke Dip (recipe follows)

3 tablespoons shredded part-skim mozzarella cheese

6 large eggs

1 teaspoon white vinegar

2 medium Roma (plum) tomatoes, sliced into thin rounds

Kosher salt and freshly ground black pepper

FOR THE DIP (3 CUPS)

1 tablespoon olive oil

1 medium onion, finely diced

1¼ teaspoons salt

3 tablespoons water

3 garlic cloves, minced

1 10-ounce package frozen chopped spinach, thawed

1 9-ounce package frozen artichoke hearts, thawed

1 cup plain nonfat Greek yogurt

3 tablespoons light mayonnaise

½ cup shredded part-skim mozzarella cheese

¼ cup finely grated Parmigiano-Reggiano cheese

2 teaspoons finely chopped fresh oregano (or 1 teaspoon dried)

½ teaspoon red pepper flakes

SERVES 6   TOTAL TIME: 45 MINUTES

1. Preheat the oven to 400°F.

2. Heat the olive oil over medium heat in a medium skillet. Add the onion and ¼ teaspoon salt and cook, stirring occasionally, until the onion begins to soften and turn translucent, 7 to 8 minutes. Add the water and garlic and continue to cook, stirring, until the onion is softened and lightly golden and the water is almost all evaporated, another 4 to 5 minutes. Transfer to a large bowl and cool for 5 minutes.

3. While the onion mixture is cooling, put the spinach and artichoke hearts on a large, clean kitchen towel and roll up the towel into a tube. Twist the ends toward each other and keep twisting until you wring out as much liquid as you can. When the vegetables are dry, chop them and add to the bowl with the onion. Add the yogurt, mayonnaise, mozzarella, Parmigiano-Reggiano cheese, oregano, remaining 1 teaspoon salt, and the red pepper flakes.

4. Prepare the toasts: Arrange the split sandwich thins on a rimmed baking sheet and spread a generous ½ cup of the dip on each half. Sprinkle each with 1½ teaspoons (½ tablespoon) of the mozzarella. Bake until the bread is toasted on the edges, the dip is cooked, and the cheese is bubbly, about 20 minutes.

continued on page 42

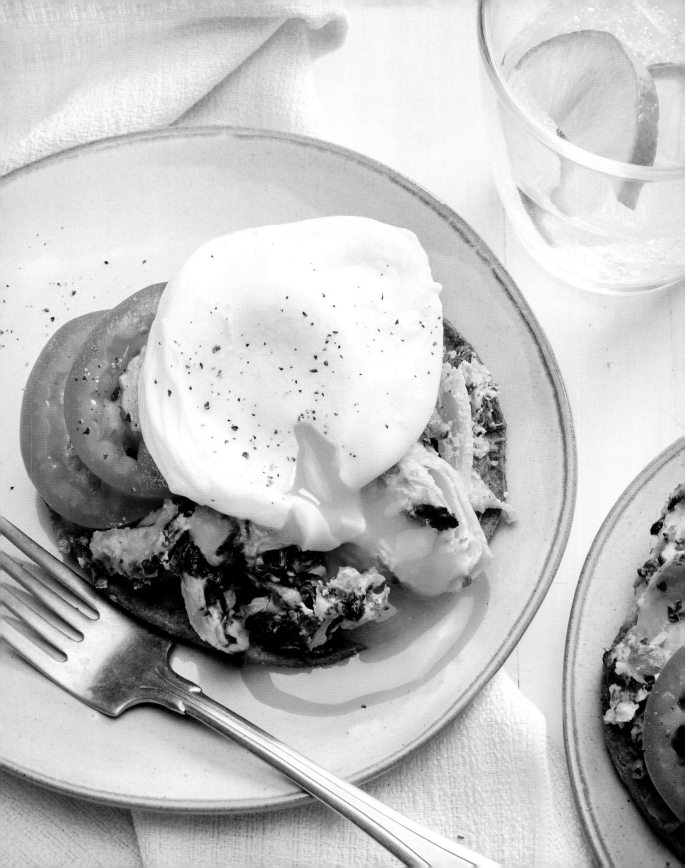

continued from page 40

5. Poach the eggs: Do this about 10 minutes before the dip is done. See the method on page 26.

6. Assemble and serve: Remove the baked toasts from the oven and arrange a few tomato slices on top of each. Season to taste with salt and pepper, then top each toast with a poached egg. Serve.

7. Note: This recipe doesn't store well. We suggest making it fresh and serving immediately.

NUTRITIONAL INFORMATION (1 SERVING = 1 EGG ON ½ SANDWICH THIN, WITH 1/2 CUP SAUCE) Calories 250, Total Fat 11.9 g 18%, Saturated Fat 3.2 g 16%, Trans Fat 0.1 g, Cholesterol 194.2 mg 65%, Sodium 833.6 mg 35%, Total Carb 21.9 g 7%, Dietary Fiber 6.2 g 25%, Sugars 4.4 g, Added Sugars 0 g, Protein 16.6 g 33%, Vitamin D 41 mcg 10%, Calcium 193.6 mg 19%, Iron 2.8 mg 15%, Potassium 469.5 mg 13%

NOOM CHEF'S TIP *Don't be afraid to try poaching an egg—it's not as difficult as you might think, and we've got some photos and instructions on page 26 to show you how. You'll feel like a master chef when you've done it. That being said, if you plan to batch-cook this recipe to make breakfasts for the week (or if you're truly anti–poached egg), you could scramble or fry the eggs instead. We've already taken liberties with the classic eggs Benedict, so you can, too.*

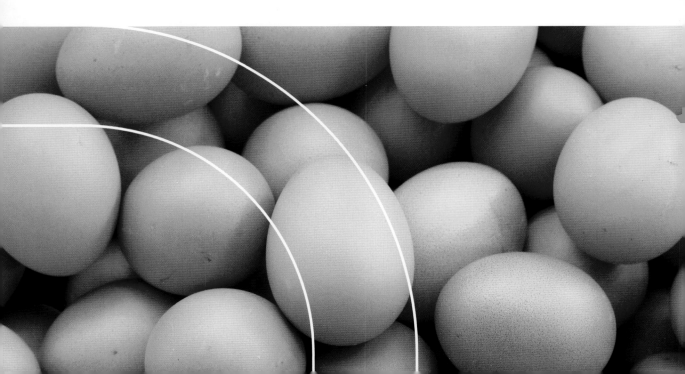

Black Bean & Quinoa Breakfast Burrito

Who doesn't love a breakfast burrito? This light version is fiber packed and protein full without any meat *or* cheese. The recipe does contain eggs and nonfat Greek yogurt, but you plant-based folks can substitute extra-firm tofu or crumbled tempeh, or just leave out the egg entirely. The quinoa has as much protein as an egg, so either way this burrito is a filling, delicious way to start your day!

¾ cup quinoa

Black Bean Filling (recipe follows)

5 large eggs plus 5 egg whites

Kosher salt

6 8-inch whole-grain tortillas

1 cup shredded iceberg lettuce

6 tablespoons plain nonfat Greek yogurt

⅔ cup diced ripe tomatoes

½ large avocado, pitted, peeled, and diced

1 cup tomatillo salsa (aka salsa verde or green salsa), for serving (store-bought, or see recipe for Chilaquiles, page 46)

BLACK BEAN FILLING

1 tablespoon olive oil

1 medium onion, finely diced

2 garlic cloves, finely minced

1 14-ounce can no-salt-added black beans, drained and rinsed

1 teaspoon ground cumin

½ teaspoon kosher salt

¼ teaspoon cayenne

¼ cup chopped fresh cilantro

SERVES 6   TOTAL TIME: 1 HOUR

1. Make the quinoa: Rinse the quinoa in a fine-mesh strainer under cold running water for 1 minute, draining the water 2 to 3 times to remove any bubbly residue.

2. Bring a medium (at least 4-quart) pot of generously salted water to a boil over high heat. (We like to add about 1 teaspoon kosher salt per quart of water.) Add the quinoa, return to a boil, and cook until the quinoa is fluffy and has popped open to display a tiny white squiggle, 18 to 20 minutes.

3. Drain well using a fine-mesh strainer, then spread out the quinoa on a rimmed baking sheet to further dry out. (You will have about 2¼ cups quinoa.)

4. Make the eggs: Whisk the eggs and egg whites in a medium bowl and add a pinch of salt. Spray a large nonstick pan with cooking spray and heat over medium-low heat. Add the eggs and cook, stirring, until fluffy, 2 to 3 minutes. Remove from the heat and cover to keep warm.

5. Make the black bean filling: Heat the olive oil in a small saucepan over medium heat. Add the onion and cook, stirring, until translucent, 6 to 7 minutes. Add the garlic and cook 1 additional minute. Add the black beans, cumin, salt, and cayenne and cook, stirring, until warmed through, 2 to 3 minutes. Stir in the cilantro and remove the pan from heat.

6. Build the burritos: Arrange a tortilla on a flat work surface. Spread about 3 tablespoons of the lettuce in a 4-by-2-inch rectangle just below the center of the tortilla. Layer on about 3 tablespoons each of the quinoa and black bean mixture, then top

continued on page 45

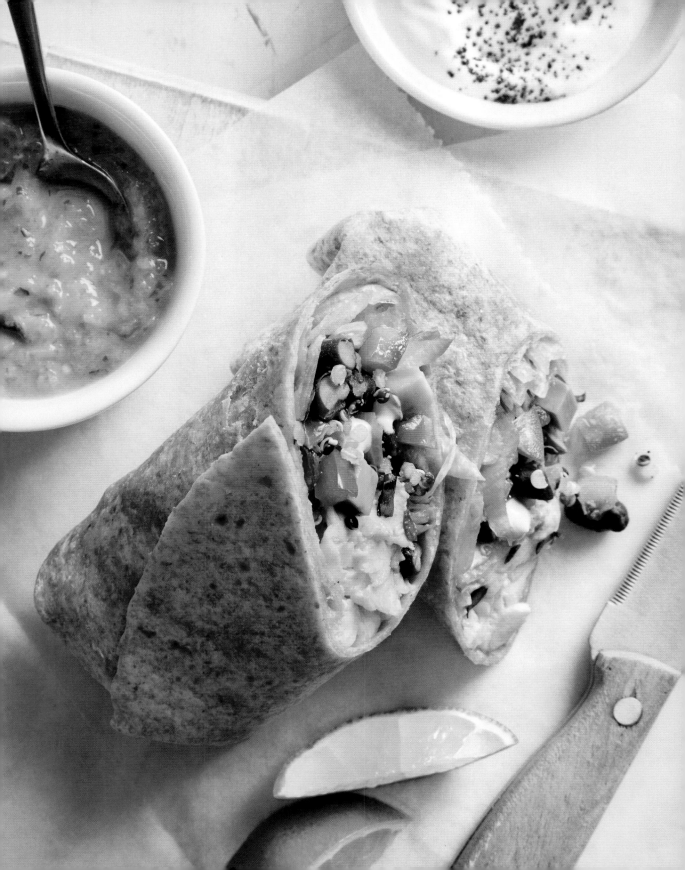

continued from page 43

with ⅙ of the egg mixture (about ⅓ cup) and about 2 tablespoons each diced tomatoes and avocado. Top with a 1-tablespoon dollop of yogurt. Pull the bottom side of the tortilla over the filling, then roll away from you, folding in the sides and then rolling tightly into a log. Repeat for the remaining 5 burritos.

7. Crisp the burritos (optional): If desired, place the burritos in a dry large (12-inch) nonstick skillet over medium heat, and crisp them, turning occasionally, until golden in parts, 2 to 3 minutes total. Serve with the salsa.

Note: If making only one burrito per day, the salsa, beans, and quinoa can all be refrigerated in airtight containers for up to 5 days.

NUTRITIONAL INFORMATION (1 SERVING = 1 BURRITO, PLUS ¼ CUP SALSA AND 1 TABLESPOON YOGURT) Calories 450, Total Fat 14.9 g 23%, Saturated Fat 2.5 g 12%, Trans Fat 0.1 g, Cholesterol 156.7 mg 52%, Sodium 681.9 mg 28%, Total Carb 58.1 g 19%, Dietary Fiber 10.4 g 42%, Sugars 6.4 g, Added Sugars 0 g, Protein 23.6 g 47%, Vitamin D 34.2 mcg 9%, Calcium 121.5 mg 12%, Iron 3.1 mg 17%, Potassium 690.4 mg 20%

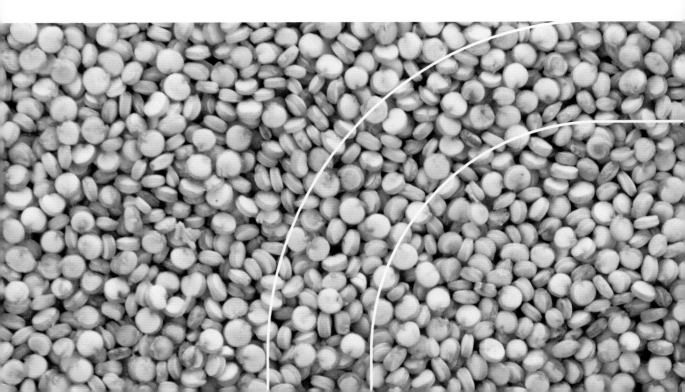

Chilaquiles

Chilaquiles are essentially corn tortilla pieces sautéed in a little oil, then simmered with salsa, cheese, beans, and eggs—although what your chilaquiles include is up to you. This version uses tangy green tomatillos instead of red salsa.

4 6-inch corn tortillas

2 teaspoons olive oil

4 large eggs

Tomatillo Salsa (recipe follows)

2 cups Black Bean Filling, warmed (see page 43), or any favorite beans

¼ cup chopped red onion

¼ cup diced avocado

¼ cup fresh cilantro leaves

FOR THE TOMATILLO SALSA

1 tablespoon olive oil

1 large onion, diced

2 garlic cloves, sliced

1 medium jalapeño, diced (and seeded, if you want less heat)

1½ cups drained canned whole tomatillos, halved (or see Chef's Tip for roasting fresh tomatillos)

⅓ cup water

½ teaspoon salt

⅓ cup chopped fresh cilantro

SERVES 4 TOTAL TIME: 45 MINUTES

1. Make the tortilla strips: Preheat the oven to 375°F.

2. Place each tortilla on a cutting board and use a pastry brush to evenly coat both sides with the olive oil.

3. Cut the tortillas into ½-inch-thick strips. Spread the strips out evenly on a rimmed baking sheet. Bake until golden and crisped, about 30 minutes, tossing them halfway through to evenly toast. (Baked tortillas can be stored for up to 5 days in an airtight container.)

4. Make the tomatillo salsa: Heat the olive oil in a medium (at least 4-quart) pot over medium-high heat. Add the onion and cook, stirring occasionally, until lightly golden, 2 minutes. Add the garlic and cook for 1 more minute.

5. Add the jalapeño, tomatillos, water, and salt to the pot. Use a potato masher or fork to carefully press down on the tomatillos to release some of their juices. Cook over medium heat until the tomatillos are completely broken down and the sauce is slightly thickened, about 5 minutes. Remove from the heat and cool slightly.

6. Make the eggs: Spray a large (12-inch) nonstick skillet with cooking spray and heat over medium heat. Crack the eggs into the skillet and cook until the whites are set but the yolks are still runny, 2 to 3 minutes.

7. Assemble the chilaquiles: Place the salsa in a large (12-inch) nonstick skillet and warm over medium-low heat until sputtering, 2 to 3 minutes. Add the tortilla strips and toss to coat.

8. Divide the tortilla mixture among 4 plates. Use a spatula to transfer 1 fried egg to top each plate, then spoon approximately ½ cup of the beans on each plate. Garnish each serving with 1 tablespoon each of the red onion, avocado, and cilantro leaves.

NUTRITIONAL INFORMATION (1 SERVING = 1 EGG, 1 TORTILLA, 1 CUP SALSA, AND ½ CUP BLACK BEANS) Calories 356, Total Fat 17.4 g 27%, Saturated Fat 3.2 g 16%, Trans Fat 0.1 g, Cholesterol 186 mg 62%, Sodium 575.6 mg 24%, Total Carb 37 g 12%, Dietary Fiber 9.2 g 37%, Sugars 5.8 g, Added Sugars 0 g, Protein 14.8 g 30%, Vitamin D 41 mcg 10%, Calcium 121.6 mg 12%, Iron 3.2 mg 18%, Potassium 642 mg 18%

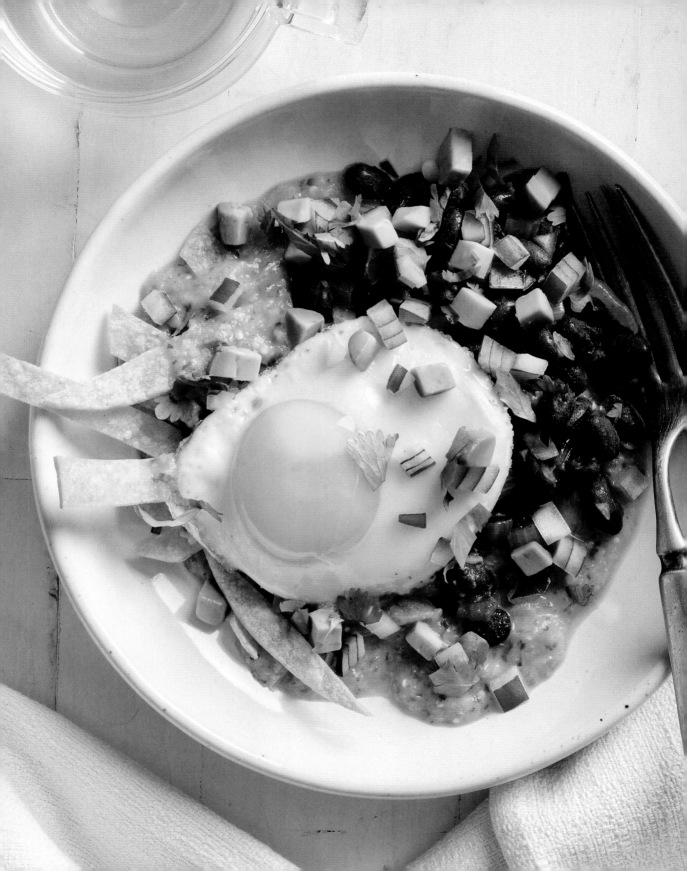

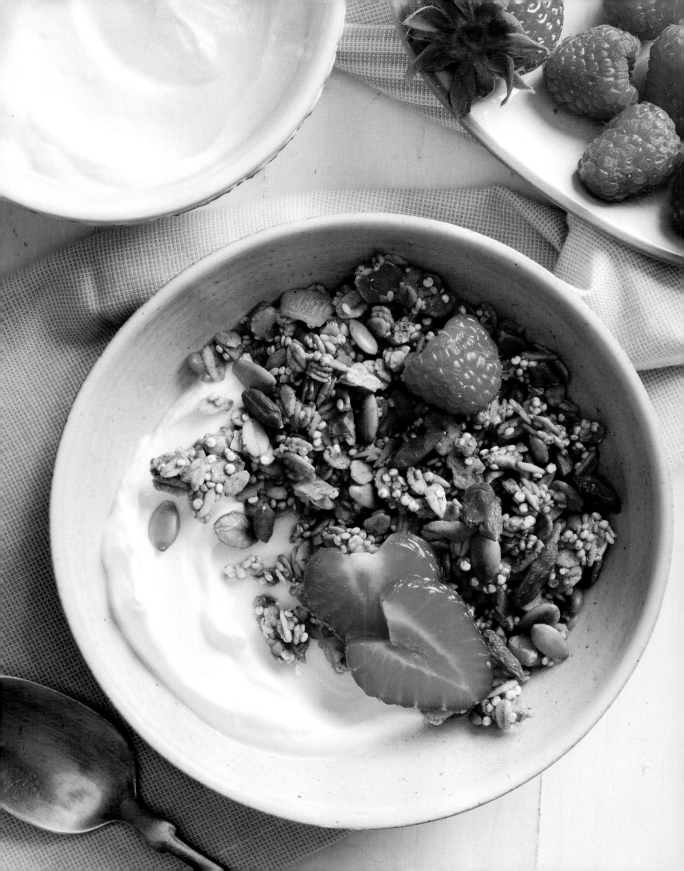

Crispy Quinoa Granola

⅔ cup quinoa

2 cups old-fashioned rolled oats

¼ cup chopped pecans

¼ cup pumpkin seeds

2 tablespoons unsweetened shredded coconut

1 tablespoon sesame seeds

¼ cup pure maple syrup

2 tablespoons coconut oil, melted

1 teaspoon vanilla extract

1 teaspoon ground cinnamon

½ teaspoon ground cardamom

¼ teaspoon kosher salt

1 large egg white

2 tablespoons dried goji berries

6 cups plain nonfat Greek yogurt

Fresh berries or other chopped fruit (optional)

Enjoy this tasty granola on nonfat Greek yogurt, as in this recipe, with or without fresh fruit, or with a simple splash of your preferred milk. Just remember that with calorically dense foods, a little goes a long way.

SERVES 12 TOTAL TIME: 35 MINUTES

1. Preheat the oven to 325°F. Line a baking sheet with parchment.

2. Mix the granola: In a large bowl, combine the quinoa, oats, pecans, pumpkin seeds, coconut, and sesame seeds.

3. Stir in the maple syrup, coconut oil, vanilla, cinnamon, cardamom, and salt until incorporated.

4. In a separate bowl, whisk the egg white until soft peaks form, 2 minutes. Gently fold into the granola.

5. Bake the granola: Spread the granola evenly on the baking sheet, and bake until it begins to become fragrant, 15 minutes. Remove from the oven, stir, return to the oven, and continue to bake until granola is toasted and crisp, about another 5 minutes.

6. Transfer the granola to a bowl and stir in the goji berries. Let the granola cool.

7. Serve the granola: Portion ⅓ cup of the granola into individual bowls, then top each serving with ½ cup of the yogurt and add the fresh fruit for garnish, if desired.

Note: You can store extra granola in an airtight container for up to 1 month.

NUTRITIONAL INFORMATION (INCLUDING YOGURT AND BERRIES) (1 SERVING = ⅓ CUP GRANOLA, PLUS ½ CUP YOGURT) Calories 308, Total Fat 9.5 g 15%, Saturated Fat 3.8 g 19%, Trans Fat 0.1 g, Cholesterol 5.7 mg 2%, Sodium 82.5 mg 3%, Total Carb 37.7 g 13%, Dietary Fiber 4.5 g 18%, Sugars 8.7 g, Added Sugars 0 g, Protein 18.9 g 38%, Vitamin D 0.0 mcg 0%, Calcium 151.3 mg 15%, Iron 2.4 mg 13%, Potassium 366.3 mg 10%

NUTRITIONAL INFORMATION (GRANOLA ONLY) (1 SERVING = ⅓ CUP GRANOLA, PLUS ½ CUP YOGURT) Calories 241, Total Fat 9.1 g 14%, Saturated Fat 3.6 g 18%, Trans Fat 0.0 g, Cholesterol 0.0 mg 0%, Sodium 41.6 mg 2%, Total Carb 33.6 g 11%, Dietary Fiber 4.5 g 18%, Sugars 5.1 g, Added Sugars 0 g, Protein 7.3 g 15%, Vitamin D 0.0 mcg 0%, Calcium 26.5 mg 3%, Iron 2.3 mg 13%, Potassium 206.2 mg 6%

Everything Bagel Avocado Toast

Everything-bagel seasoning is one of our favorite flavors, especially on this quick avocado toast with pickled onion. Pickling is surprisingly easy—just mix the marinade, cook it with the onion, and let it soak briefly. Voilà! You made your own fancy condiment. Be proud!

FOR THE PICKLED RED ONION

1½ cups apple cider vinegar

1 tablespoon sugar

5 whole black peppercorns

1 bay leaf

½ teaspoon kosher salt

1 large red onion, sliced into thin rings

FOR THE TOASTS

1 small avocado, halved, pitted, and peeled

2½-inch-thick slices whole-grain sourdough bread, toasted until golden

2 teaspoons everything-bagel seasoning

Flaky sea salt, such as Maldon

SERVES 2   TOTAL TIME: 50 MINUTES (INCLUDING PICKLING THE ONION)

1. Make the pickled red onion: In a small saucepan over medium-high heat, bring the vinegar, sugar, peppercorns, bay leaf, and salt to a boil. Add the onion and cook for 1 minute. Remove from the heat and let the onion rest in the liquid for 10 minutes.

2. Drain and reserve the liquid. Place the onion in a small bowl. Let the onion and liquid separately cool to room temperature (this keeps the onion from getting mushy).

3. Place the onion in a small jar, cover with the liquid, seal the jar, and refrigerate until chilled, about 30 minutes. (You can keep the pickled onion refrigerated in an airtight container for up to 1 month.)

4. Assemble the toasts and serve: Arrange the avocado halves cut side down on a cutting board. Use a thin, sharp knife to thinly slice the avocado halves, then gently press the slices to fan them out.

5. Put the toasts on 2 individual plates, then carefully transfer half the sliced avocado onto each toast—a spatula can help keep the avocado halves in their pretty, fanned-out pattern.

6. Arrange 1 to 2 tablespoons of drained pickled onion on top of each avocado toast, then sprinkle each with 1 teaspoon bagel seasoning. (If your bagel seasoning doesn't contain salt, garnish with flaky sea salt; if it does contain salt, skip this step.) Serve.

NUTRITIONAL INFORMATION (1 SERVING = 1 TOAST) Calories 268, Total Fat 10.8 g 17%, Saturated Fat 1.4 g 7%, Trans Fat 0.0 g, Cholesterol 0.0 mg 0%, Sodium 401.1 mg 17%, Total Carb 32.6 g 11%, Dietary Fiber 8.6 g 34%, Sugars 6.2 g, Added Sugars 0 g, Protein 8.4 g 17%, Vitamin D 0.0 mcg 0%, Calcium 53 mg 5%, Iron 1.6 mg 9%, Potassium 359.1 mg 10%

NOOM CHEF'S TIP: FURIKAKE *This recipe is great for experimenting with different flavor profiles. Instead of the everything-bagel seasoning, you could use Japanese furikake—a savory combination of sesame, seaweed, and spices. It pairs amazingly with the avocado and pickled onion.*

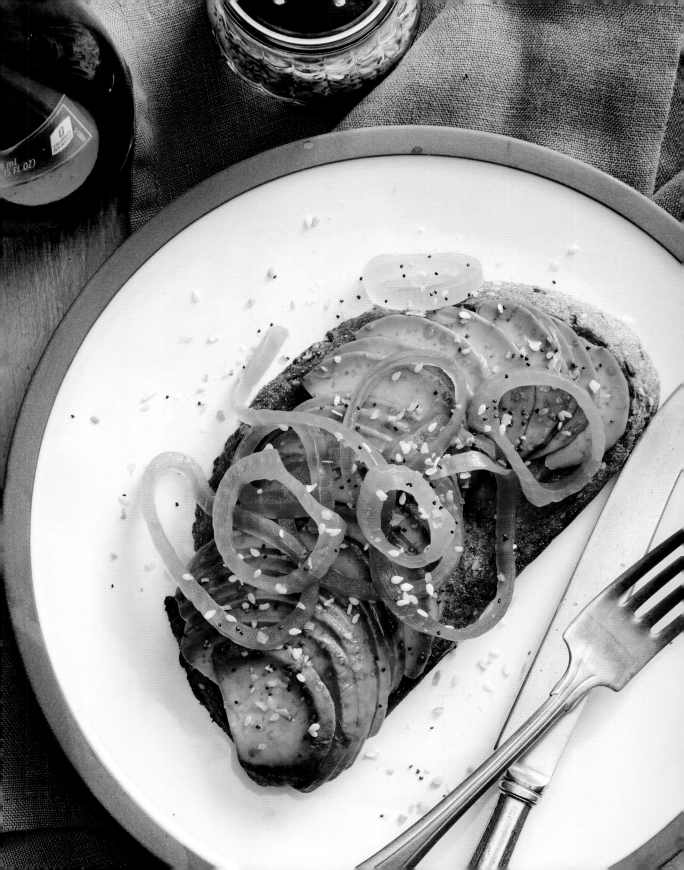

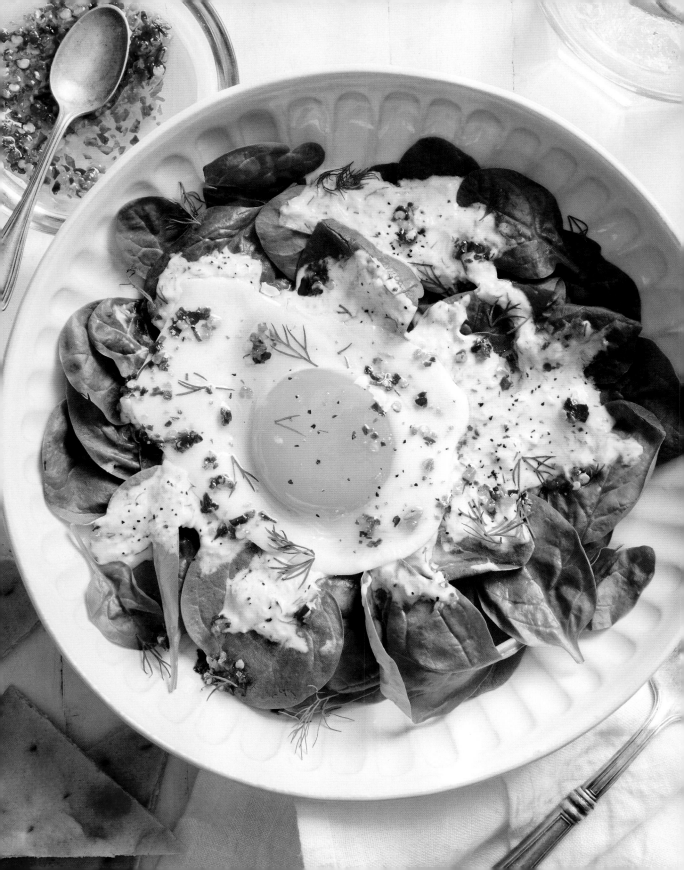

Garlicky Eggs with Chili Oil

If you want to make this recipe even more Noom-ish, you can serve it over a bed of spinach or other cooked veggies. If you really like this sauce, you can double the recipe and use it as a salad dressing, a dip, or a drizzle. This tasty sauce is truly versatile.

Traditionally the eggs are poached, but we adapted this one using a fried egg instead. Of course, if you are into tradition, you can keep practicing your egg-poaching skills with this recipe—check out our how-to guide on page 26.

FOR THE YOGURT

1 medium Persian cucumber (or 3-inch piece English cucumber)

1 cup plain nonfat Greek yogurt

2 tablespoons chopped fresh dill

2 garlic cloves, very finely minced

¼ teaspoon kosher salt

FOR THE CHILI OIL

1 tablespoon olive oil

1 teaspoon unsalted butter

1 garlic clove, very finely minced

½ teaspoon red pepper flakes, or more to taste

Kosher salt

FOR THE EGGS AND SERVING

2 large eggs

Chopped fresh dill

Kosher salt and freshly ground black pepper

SERVES 2   TOTAL TIME: 15 MINUTES

1. Make the yogurt: Grate the cucumber into a medium bowl, then add the yogurt, dill, garlic, and salt. Let the yogurt mixture sit at room temperature until you're ready to use it.

2. Make the chili oil: Combine the olive oil, butter, garlic, red pepper flakes, and a pinch of salt in a microwave-safe ramekin, leaving a couple inches of headroom. Microwave on high for 60 seconds, remove from the microwave, and stir, then microwave for an additional 30 seconds, or until fragrant, toasty looking, and the garlic has softened.

3. Fry the eggs: Coat a large (12-inch) nonstick skillet with cooking spray and place over medium-high heat. Add the eggs and fry to desired doneness.

4. Serve the dish: Divide the yogurt mixture between 2 serving plates, then arrange a fried egg on top of each bed of yogurt. Stir the chili oil and drizzle it over the eggs, dividing it between the 2 plates. Garnish each plate with some dill and season to taste with salt and pepper.

NUTRITIONAL INFORMATION (SERVING = 1 CUP SPINACH, 1 EGG, ⅔ CUP YOGURT MIXTURE, AND 1 TABLESPOON CHILI OIL) Calories 245, Total Fat 14.2 g 22%, Saturated Fat 3.9 g 19%, Trans Fat 0.2 g, Cholesterol 196.8 mg 66%, Sodium 543.2 mg 23%, Total Carb 11.3 g 4%, Dietary Fiber 1.2 g 5%, Sugars 4.8 g, Added Sugars 0 g, Protein 19.7 g 39%, Vitamin D 42.4 mcg 11%, Calcium 280.9 mg 28%, Iron 4.2 mg 24%, Potassium 528.5 mg 15%

NOOM CHEF'S TIP *If you know you'll be short on time, you could make the yogurt sauce up to 3 days in advance. Store it covered in the refrigerator, then let it come to room temperature before serving.*

Four-Way Rainbow Smoothies

You might be surprised by some of the ingredients in these four rainbow-bright smoothies. Cauliflower? Beets? Kale? Tahini? The beauty of these smoothies extends beyond their vibrant colors. These unusual ingredients add fiber and vitamins, helping to make the smoothies nutritious and filling. They're made with inexpensive foods you probably already have on hand, and the colors mean eating the rainbow has never been easier.

EACH SMOOTHIE SERVES 2 (1 SERVING = VARIABLE) **TOTAL TIME:** 10 MINUTES

1. To make each of these smoothies, combine the ingredients in a blender and blend until smooth.

Coconut Paradise

(1 SERVING = 1¼ CUPS)

1½ cups natural coconut water

⅔ cup frozen pineapple chunks

½ frozen banana, cut into chunks (see Chef's Tip on page 56)

10 fresh mint leaves

2 tablespoons coconut milk

½ teaspoon vanilla extract

Dash of kosher salt

NUTRITIONAL INFORMATION Calories 126, Total Fat 4.1 g 6%, Saturated Fat 3.5 g 18%, Trans Fat 0.0 g, Cholesterol 0.0 mg 0%, Sodium 264.9 mg 11%, Total Carb 21.6 g 7%, Dietary Fiber 3.9 g 15%, Sugars 14.4 g, Added Sugars 0 g, Protein 2.2 g 4%, Vitamin D 0.0 mcg 0%, Calcium 54.4 mg 5%, Iron 1 mg 6%, Potassium 656.6 mg 19%

Strawberry Blush

(1 SERVING = 1½ CUPS)

1 cup unsweetened almond milk

1 cup frozen strawberries

1 5-ounce block soft silken tofu

½ cup diced cooked beets (see Note)

½ cup frozen dark sweet cherries

2 teaspoons chia seeds

2 teaspoons ground flax seeds

½ teaspoon vanilla extract

Dash of kosher salt

Note: You can find vacuum-packed cooked beets in the produce department of some grocery stores, or you can cook your own. In a pinch, you could substitute canned beets.

NUTRITIONAL INFORMATION Calories 193, Total Fat 6.5 g 10%, Saturated Fat 0.7 g 3%, Trans Fat 0.1 g, Cholesterol 0.0 mg 0%, Sodium 203 mg 8%, Total Carb 28.5 g 9%, Dietary Fiber 6.7 g 27%, Sugars 17 g, Added Sugars 0 g, Protein 7.1 g 14%, Vitamin D 0.0 mcg 0%, Calcium 193 mg 19%, Iron 2.4 mg 13%, Potassium 525.3 mg 15%

continued on page 56

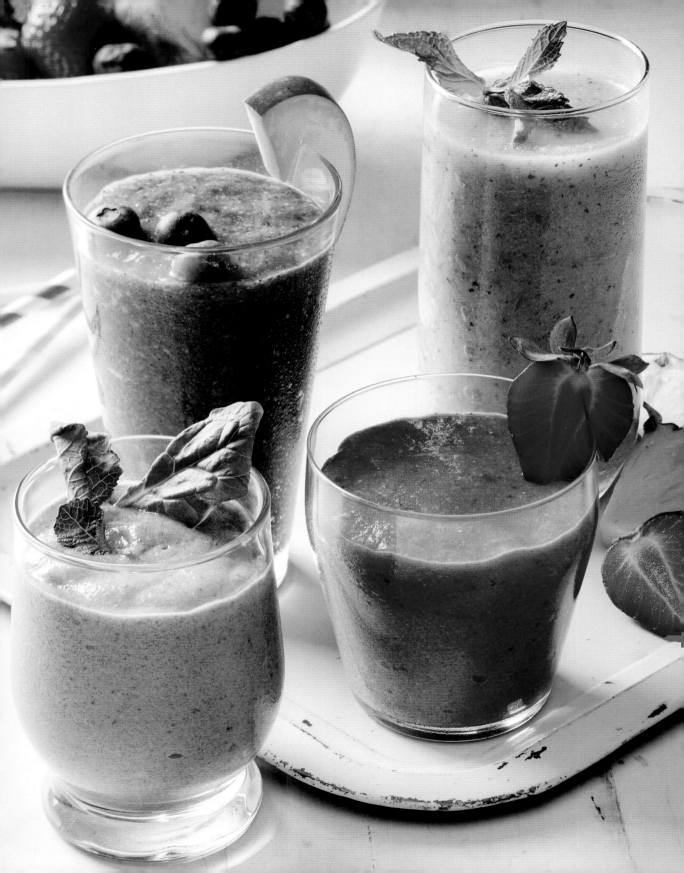

continued from page 54

● TropicBerry Delight

(1 SERVING = 1 CUP)

1½ cups unsweetened almond milk

1 cup frozen mango chunks

1 cup frozen blueberries

½ cup frozen (or fresh) cauliflower florets, thawed

2 teaspoons chia seeds

2 teaspoons ground flax seeds

½ teaspoon vanilla extract

Dash of kosher salt

NUTRITIONAL INFORMATION Calories 168, Total Fat 6 g 9%, Saturated Fat 0.5 g 2%, Trans Fat 0.1 g, Cholesterol 0.0 mg 0%, Sodium 218.2 mg 9%, Total Carb 26.3 g 9%, Dietary Fiber 7.3 g 29%, Sugars 16.9 g, Added Sugars 0 g, Protein 3.7 g 7%, Vitamin D 0.0 mcg 0%, Calcium 214.9 mg 21%, Iron 0.9 mg 5%, Potassium 377.3 mg 11%

● Green Goodness

(1 SERVING = 1¾ CUPS)

1 cup unsweetened almond milk

1 frozen banana, cut into chunks (see Chef's Tip)

2½ cups (packed) baby spinach leaves

1 cup (packed) coarsely chopped kale leaves

2 tablespoons tahini

½ teaspoon matcha powder

Dash of kosher salt

NUTRITIONAL INFORMATION Calories 196, Total Fat 10 g 15%, Saturated Fat 1.2 g 6%, Trans Fat 0.0 g, Cholesterol 0.0 mg 0%, Sodium 224.9 mg 9%, Total Carb 23.7 g 8%, Dietary Fiber 6.5 g 26%, Sugars 8 g, Added Sugars 0 g, Protein 6.5 g 13%, Vitamin D 0.0 mcg 0%, Calcium 278.8 mg 28%, Iron 4.3 mg 24%, Potassium 518.1 mg 15%,

---

NOOM CHEF'S TIP *Peel your bananas before freezing them—it's hard to peel a frozen banana!*

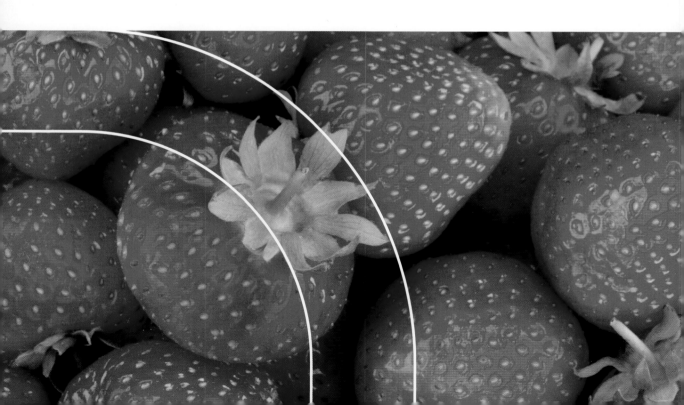

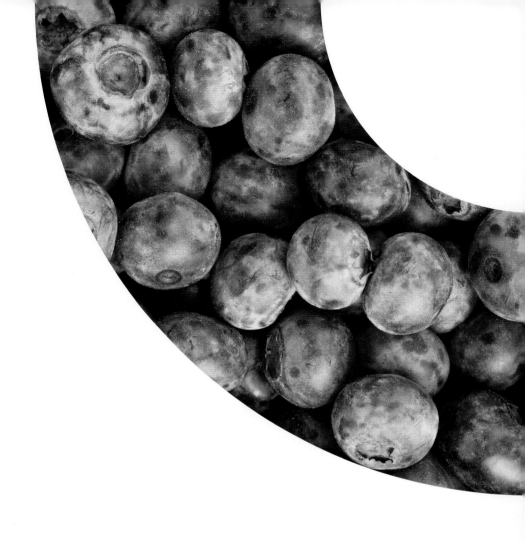

Soups and Salads

Noomers love soups and salads—soup is the ultimate comfort food, and salad is an easy and tasty way to get in lots of veggies. Both are filling, with high nutritional density and low caloric density (with the exception of really rich, creamy soups and salad dressings). All the soups and salads in this chapter are low in caloric density, so enjoy! Lip-smacking and slurping are encouraged.

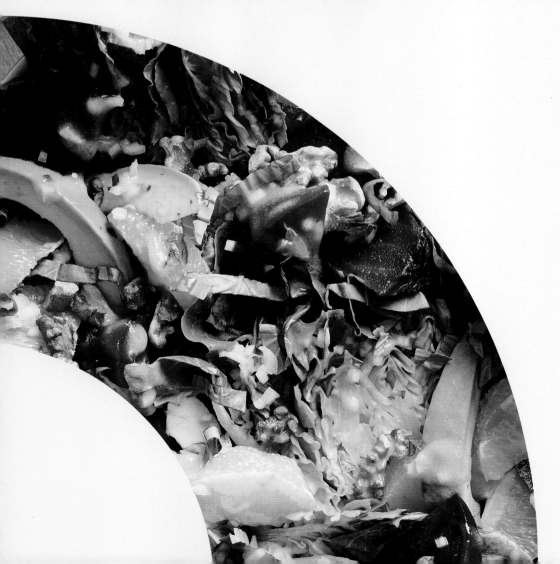

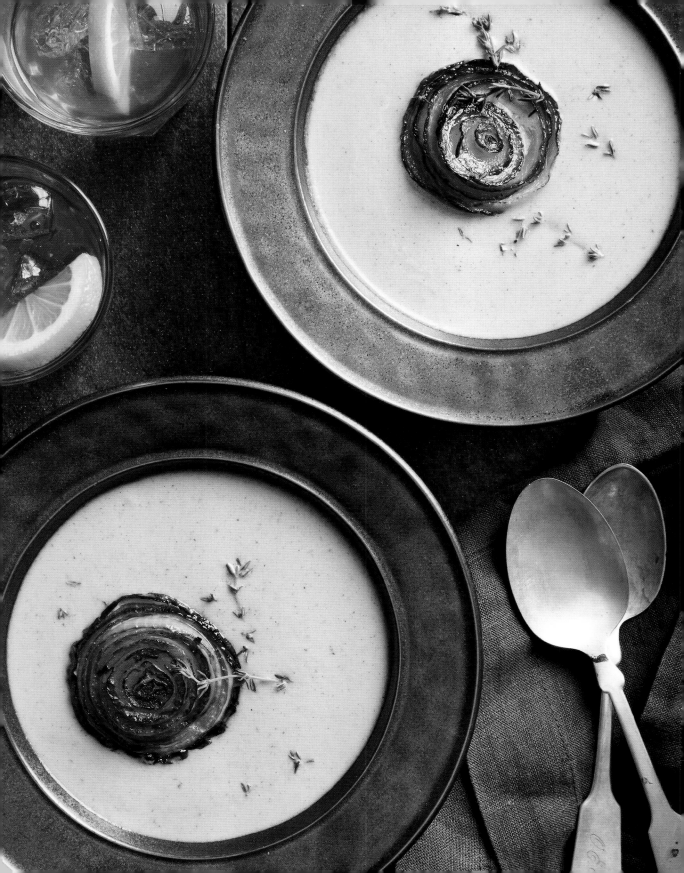

Creamy
Onion Soup

This light and creamy onion soup gets its texture from oat or almond milk. Or, if you want a more indulgent treat, you could stir in a little half-and-half at the end to enrich the soup. Either way, this oniony soup is delicious and satisfying, especially with its roasted onion rings on top. Impress your friends, impress yourself.

SERVES 4 TOTAL TIME: 1 HOUR

7 large onions

2 tablespoons olive oil

1 tablespoon thyme leaves (or 1½ teaspoons dried), plus more for garnish

2 teaspoons kosher salt, plus more for seasoning

½ teaspoon freshly ground black pepper, plus more for seasoning

1 or 2 fresh thyme sprigs

4 cups low-sodium chicken or vegetable broth

1 teaspoon unsalted butter

1 cup plain unsweetened oat or almond milk

1. Sauté the onions: Chop 6 of the onions (to make about 6 cups of chopped onions).

2. Heat 1 tablespoon of the olive oil in a large (at least 6-quart) soup pot over high heat. Add the chopped onions, the thyme leaves, 1½ teaspoons of the salt, and the pepper. Cook, stirring, until the onions begin to soften, about 10 minutes.

3. Reduce the heat to low and continue to cook the onions until they are golden and caramelized, stirring often to prevent them from burning and sticking to the pot, adding 1 to 2 tablespoons of water as needed. This should take 30 to 35 minutes.

4. Roast the onion rings: Preheat the oven to 375°F.

5. Peel the remaining onion and cut it into four ½-inch rounds. Line a baking sheet with parchment paper. Brush both sides of the onion rounds with the remaining 1 tablespoon olive oil and season generously with salt and pepper; scatter on the thyme sprigs. Roast the onion rounds until tender and golden, 30 to 35 minutes. Discard the thyme sprigs.

6. Make it soup: Add the broth to the pot with the onions, then add the butter and remaining ½ teaspoon salt. Bring the soup to a boil over high heat, reduce the heat to medium. and simmer until the onions have absorbed a bit of the liquid, about 10 minutes.

7. Add the milk and stir to incorporate, then use an immersion blender to puree until smooth (or transfer in batches to a stand blender or food processor), 30 to 45 seconds. Season to taste with more salt and pepper.

8. Serve the soup: Divide the soup among 4 bowls, top each bowl with a roasted onion round, then garnish with the remaining thyme leaves. Serve hot.

NUTRITIONAL INFORMATION (1 SERVING = 1⅔ CUPS) Calories 226, Total Fat 10.6 g 16%, Saturated Fat 2.4 g 12%, Trans Fat 0.1 g, Cholesterol 4.1 mg 1%, Sodium 864.5 mg 36%, Total Carb 27.9 g 9%, Dietary Fiber 4.6 g 18%, Sugars 11.4 g, Added Sugars 0 g, Protein 8.1 g 16%, Vitamin D 1 mcg 0%, Calcium 191.1 mg 19%, Iron 1.3 mg 7%, Potassium 612 mg 17%

Italian Wedding Soup

2 medium carrots, diced

1 medium celery stalk, sliced

6 cups low-sodium chicken broth

½ teaspoon salt

¼ teaspoon freshly ground black pepper

Italian Wedding Soup Meatballs (recipe follows)

3 cups lightly packed baby spinach leaves

2 tablespoons shredded Parmigiano-Reggiano cheese

2 tablespoons finely chopped fresh parsley

FOR THE MEATBALLS (MAKES 36)

1 tablespoon olive oil

1 large onion, finely diced

6 garlic cloves, minced

12 ounces ground white-meat chicken

1 large egg yolk

2 tablespoons nutritional yeast

¼ cup finely shredded carrot

2 tablespoons finely chopped fresh parsley

⅛ teaspoon kosher salt

¼ teaspoon freshly ground black pepper

⅛ to ¼ teaspoon red pepper flakes

One somewhat surprising ingredient that gives these meatballs their delicious taste is nutritional yeast. This flaky, cheesy-tasting condiment contains lots of B vitamins and other nutrients. It's a staple in plant-based diets, but omnivores can enjoy its taste and benefits. It's also great on popcorn.

SERVES 6   TOTAL TIME: 50 MINUTES

1. Make the meatballs: Heat the olive oil in a large (12-inch) skillet over medium heat. Add the onion and cook, stirring, until translucent and soft, 8 to 9 minutes. Add the garlic and cook, stirring, 1 more minute.

2. Transfer to a large bowl, cool slightly, then remove half the mixture (about ⅓ cup) to a small bowl and reserve for the soup.

3. To the large bowl, add the chicken, egg yolk, and nutritional yeast and stir until combined. Add the shredded carrot, parsley, salt, pepper, and red pepper flakes. Gently mix with your hands to incorporate.

4. Line a baking sheet with parchment paper. Form meatballs, using 1½ to 2 teaspoons of the mixture per ball. Set the sheet aside while you make the broth.

5. Make it soup: Transfer the reserved onion mixture to a medium (at least 4-quart) saucepan. Add the diced carrots and celery and cook over medium heat until the carrots begin to soften, 2 to 3 minutes.

6. Add the broth, salt, and pepper. Bring the soup to a boil, then simmer until the vegetables are tender, about 10 minutes.

7. Using a slotted spoon or fork, gently lower the meatballs into the soup, occasionally stirring so they don't stick together. Bring the soup to a boil over high heat, then lower the heat to medium-low and simmer until the meatballs are cooked through and the soup has darkened slightly, 8 to 10 minutes. During the last 3 minutes of simmering, add the spinach leaves.

8. Garnish and serve the soup: Divide the soup among 6 bowls, and garnish each bowl with 1 teaspoon of Parmigiano-Reggiano. Sprinkle the parsley over the tops and serve hot.

NUTRITIONAL INFORMATION (1 SERVING = 1 GENEROUS CUP BROTH, WITH 6 MINI MEATBALLS) Calories 155, Total Fat 5.7 g 9%, Saturated Fat 1.3 g 6%, Trans Fat 0.0 g, Cholesterol 64.2 mg 21%, Sodium 395.3 mg 16%, Total Carb 7.2 g 2%, Dietary Fiber 1.3 g 5%, Sugars 1.4 g, Added Sugars 0 g, Protein 20.3 g 41%, Vitamin D 6.2 mcg 2%, Calcium 59.9 mg 6%, Iron 1.7 mg 9%, Potassium 388 mg 11%

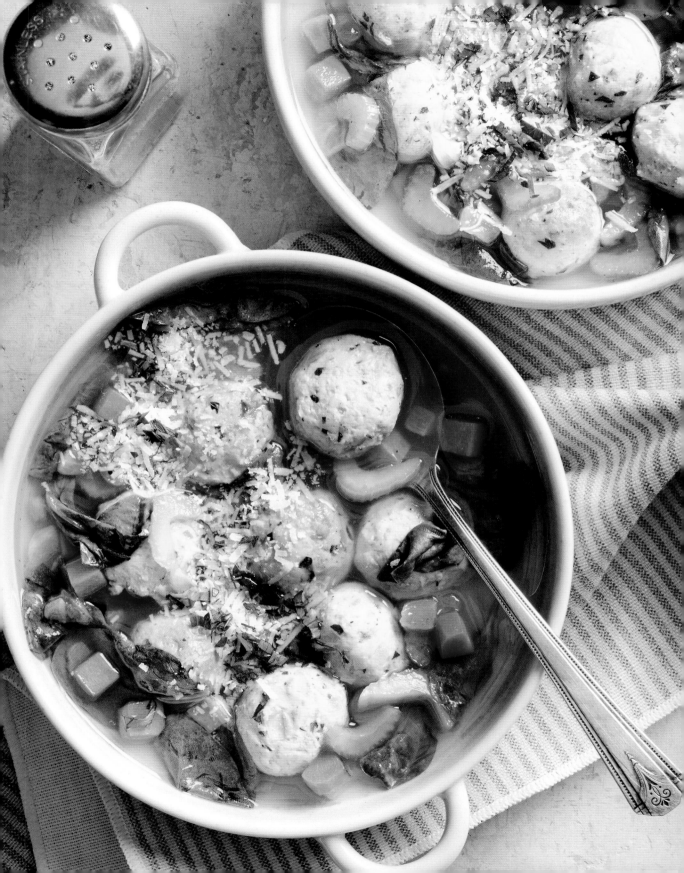

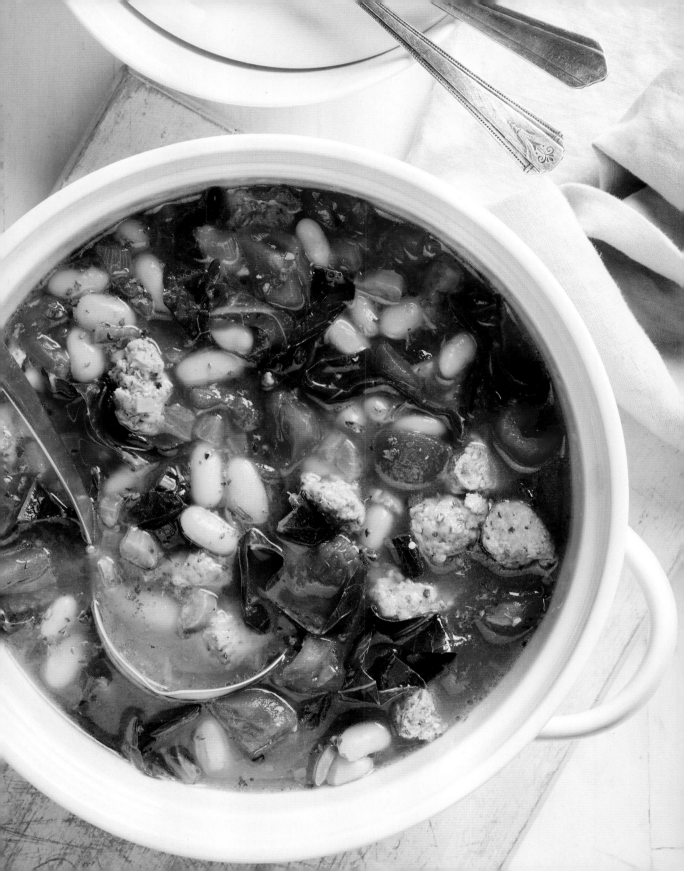

White Bean & Sausage Soup

12 ounces Swiss chard

1 tablespoon olive oil

8 ounces hot or sweet Italian-flavored turkey sausage, crumbled

1 large onion, finely diced

2 garlic cloves, minced

6 cups low-sodium chicken broth

1 14-ounce can cannellini beans, drained and rinsed

1 14-ounce can diced tomatoes

1 teaspoon kosher salt

1 teaspoon dried oregano

1 teaspoon dried basil

Rich with spicy sausage and hearty white beans, this soup will make you long for cozy winter days—but you can enjoy it all year round! You can use kale if you prefer, but the Swiss chard adds a pretty hue with its red stems. Those stems are edible, so you don't need to throw them out (thrifty!); the leaves are more tender than some leafy greens, like kale and collards.

Like many rich and hearty soups, this one tastes even better reheated the next day, so make enough for leftovers!

SERVES 8   TOTAL TIME: 1 HOUR

1. Prepare the chard: Separate the chard leaves from the stems. Trim the tough ends from the bottoms of the stems, then thinly slice the stems. Roll the chard leaves into a log, then slice them into ½-inch-thick ribbons.

2. Cook the sausage: Heat the olive oil in a large (about 6-quart) pot or Dutch oven over medium-high heat.

3. Add the sausage and cook, stirring and breaking up any large pieces, until evenly browned, 5 to 6 minutes. Transfer to a bowl to cool.

4. Cook the chard: Add the onion and chard stems to the pot and cook over medium-high heat, stirring up any browned bits from the bottom of the pot, until lightly golden, 8 to 9 minutes. Add the garlic and cook, stirring, 1 more minute. Add the chard greens and cook, stirring, until they are wilted but still bright green, about 3 minutes.

5. Make it soup: Return the sausage to the pot, then add the broth, beans, tomatoes and their juice, salt, oregano, and basil. Bring to a boil over medium-high heat, then reduce to medium-low and simmer, stirring occasionally, until the soup thickens slightly, 25 to 30 minutes.

6. Serve the soup: Ladle the soup into 8 individual bowls and serve.

NUTRITIONAL INFORMATION (1 SERVING = 1⅓ CUPS) Calories 152, Total Fat 5.4 g 8%, Saturated Fat 1.2 g 6%, Trans Fat 0.0 g, Cholesterol 24.7 mg 8%, Sodium 777.5 mg 32%, Total Carb 16.6 g 6%, Dietary Fiber 4.2 g 17%, Sugars 3.1 g, Added Sugars 0 g, Protein 12.7 g 25%, Vitamin D 0.0 mcg 0%, Calcium 85.7 mg 9%, Iron 4.2 mg 23%, Potassium 455.7 mg 13%

Ultimate Vegetable Soup

2 tablespoons olive oil

1 medium onion, chopped

3 garlic cloves, minced

½ pound white button mushrooms, trimmed and thinly sliced

2 medium zucchini, diced

2 large carrots, diced

1 large celery stalk, cut into thin slices

1 teaspoon kosher salt, plus more for seasoning

1 teaspoon dried oregano

1 teaspoon dried thyme

¼ teaspoon freshly ground black pepper, plus more for seasoning

6 cups low-sodium vegetable broth

1 28-ounce can diced tomatoes

1 15-ounce can chickpeas, drained and rinsed

1 bay leaf

1 Parmesan rind (optional)

4 cups raw baby spinach leaves, stems removed, leaves coarsely chopped

There's vegetable soup, and then there's *vegetable* soup. That's what this recipe is all about. It positively brims with onion, mushrooms, zucchini, celery, spinach, tomatoes, and (surprise!) chickpeas! The Parmesan rind adds a depth of flavor that will have everybody wondering what your secret is. This is no mere side dish; this soup is a real meal.

SERVES 8   TOTAL TIME: 1 HOUR 15 MINUTES

1. Sauté the vegetables: Heat the olive oil in a large (at least 6-quart) pot over medium heat. Add the onion and cook, stirring, until lightly golden, 8 to 9 minutes. Add the garlic and cook 1 more minute. Add the mushrooms and cook, stirring, until they release their water and soften, 5 to 6 minutes.

2. Add the zucchini, carrots, celery, salt, oregano, thyme, and pepper and cook, stirring, until the vegetables begin to soften, about 5 minutes.

3. Make it soup: Add the vegetable broth, tomatoes with their juices, chickpeas, bay leaf, and Parmesan rind if using. Bring to a boil, reduce the heat to a medium-low, and simmer, partially covered and stirring occasionally, until the soup thickens slightly, about 45 minutes. Stir in the spinach and cook an additional 5 minutes.

4. Serve the soup: Remove the Parmesan rind and bay leaf, then season the soup to taste with additional salt and pepper. Divide among 8 bowls and serve.

Note: This soup is even better the next day.

NUTRITIONAL INFORMATION (1 SERVING = 2 CUPS) Calories 138, Total Fat 4.5 g 7%, Saturated Fat 0.6 g 3%, Trans Fat 0.0 g, Cholesterol 0.0 mg 0%, Sodium 623.6 mg 26%, Total Carb 20.5 g 7%, Dietary Fiber 5.4 g 22%, Sugars 6.9 g, Added Sugars 0 g, Protein 5.2 g 10%, Vitamin D 2 mcg 0%, Calcium 77.8 mg 8%, Iron 2 mg 11%, Potassium 326.8 mg 9%

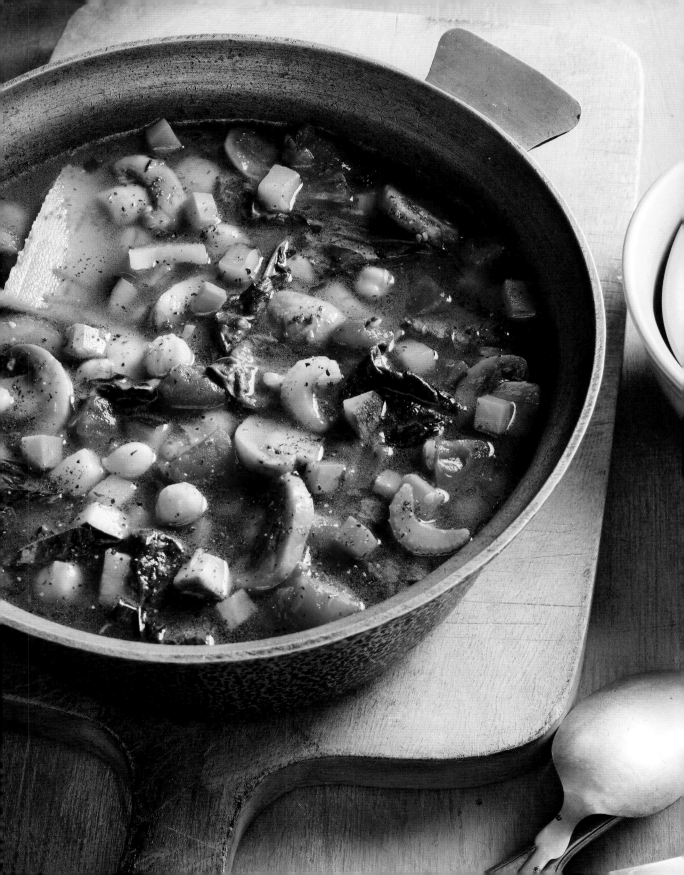

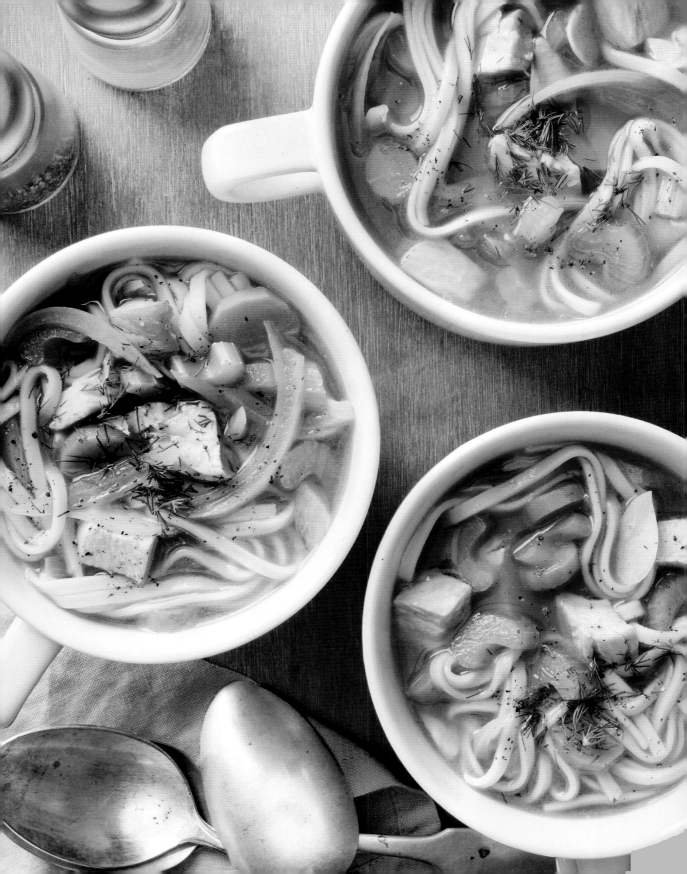

Not-Quite-Classic Chicken Noodle Soup

Is there anything more comforting in the middle of winter, or when you're home sick with the sniffles? But—what's this about shirataki noodles? Just wait until you hear! These have been called "miracle noodles." They have no carbs, and hardly any calories. The kind of fiber they contain is great for digestion, and people who avoid gluten can enjoy all the shirataki noodles they want. The noodles are found in the refrigerator case of many grocery stores, or you can buy vacuum-sealed packages online.

1 pound boneless, skinless chicken breasts (about 2 large)

1 teaspoon kosher salt, plus more for seasoning

2 tablespoons olive oil

1 large onion, halved and sliced into half-moons

3 garlic cloves, sliced

4 medium carrots, cut into ½-inch rounds

3 celery stalks, sliced

8 cups chicken broth

2 7- to 8-ounce packages fettuccine-style shirataki (or shirataki-tofu blend) noodles

1 teaspoon fresh lemon juice

Chopped fresh dill

SERVES 6   TOTAL TIME: 55 MINUTES

1. Cook the chicken: Pat the chicken breasts dry and season with ½ teaspoon salt.

2. Heat 1 tablespoon of the olive oil in a medium (4-quart) saucepan over medium heat. Place the chicken breasts in the pot, cover and steam-sear, making sure not to burn, until the undersides of the chicken are golden but not deeply browned, 5 to 6 minutes.

3. Flip the breasts and cook until the other side is golden but not deeply browned, another 5 to 6 minutes. Transfer the chicken to a plate and let cool briefly. Cut into ½-inch cubes.

4. Sauté the vegetables: Add the remaining tablespoon oil to the pot, set over medium-low heat, and add the onion. Cook, stirring frequently, until the onion is lightly golden, 6 to 7 minutes.

5. Add the garlic and cook, stirring, about 1 minute. Add the carrots, celery, and remaining ½ teaspoon salt. Increase the heat to medium and cook, stirring, until the carrots begin to soften, 3 to 4 minutes.

6. Make it soup: Add the broth to the pot and increase the heat to high. Bring to a boil, reduce the heat to medium-low, and simmer, partially covered, until the vegetables are tender and the broth has deepened slightly in color, 20 to 25 minutes, stirring occasionally.

7. Soak the noodles: While the soup is simmering, drain the noodles in a colander, rinse them well, and drain again. Put them in a medium bowl with the lemon juice and toss to coat. Let the noodles stand for 2 minutes, then rinse and drain again (this improves the taste and texture of the noodles).

continued on page 70

continued from page 69

8. Complete the soup and serve: Return the chicken and any accumulated juices to the pot and add the noodles. Cook until just warmed through, 3 to 4 minutes. Season to taste with more salt, if desired. Divide the soup among 6 bowls and garnish with the dill. Serve while still hot.

NUTRITIONAL INFORMATION (1 SERVING = GENEROUS 2 CUPS) Calories 180, Total Fat 7.2 g 11%, Saturated Fat 1.1 g 5%, Trans Fat 0.0 g, Cholesterol 48.4 mg 16%, Sodium 1618.7 mg 67%, Total Carb 10.4 g 3%, Dietary Fiber 3.8 g 15%, Sugars 3.8 g, Added Sugars 0 g, Protein 19.2 g 38%, Vitamin D 3.8 mcg 1%, Calcium 113.5 mg 11%, Iron 2.8 mg 16%, Potassium 612.3 mg 17%

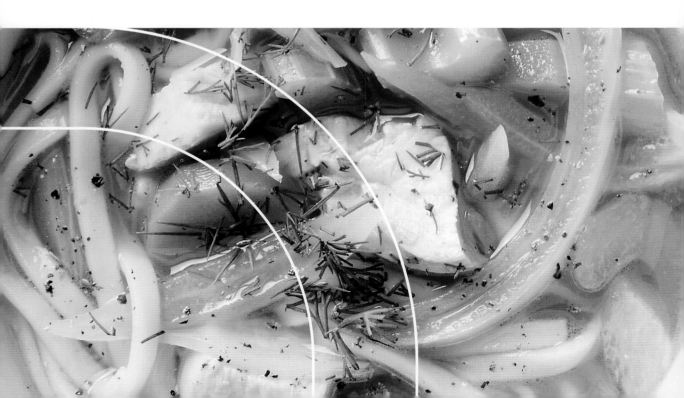

Kicky Cauliflower-Leek Soup

1 small head cauliflower

1 large leek

2 tablespoons olive oil

3 garlic cloves, minced

5 cups low-sodium vegetable or chicken broth

1 teaspoon kosher salt

Generous pinch of grated nutmeg

¼ cup sunflower seeds

⅛ teaspoon cayenne

2 tablespoons thinly sliced scallion greens

We love creamy soups, but we don't love how calorically dense they can be. Not this version, though! The creaminess in this blended soup comes from the cauliflower, and the leek gives the soup a unique savory quality that is a little milder and sweeter than regular onion. Leeks are also known to help your body get rid of excess fluid.

SERVES 4 TOTAL TIME: 55 MINUTES (INCLUDING CHILLING)

1. Prepare the cauliflower and leeks: Remove the bottom leaves and core the cauliflower head. Separate the florets and cut them short, then slice the remaining parts of the stems into ½-inch-thick pieces; you should have about 5 cups total florets and stems.

2. Trim about ½ inch from the top of the leek and discard. Trim the roots. Using a sharp paring knife, cut halfway through the leek lengthwise until you reach the center of the white part (leek will remain intact).

3. Run the leek under cold water, exposing the layers to remove any sand. Drain well and thinly slice the leek crosswise, starting with the green leaves. Discard the root end.

4. Sauté the vegetables: Heat the olive oil in a medium to large (at least 4-quart) saucepan over medium heat. Add the leek, lower the heat to medium-low, and cook, stirring occasionally, until the leek softens but doesn't darken, 6 to 8 minutes. Add the garlic and cook, stirring, until fragrant, about 1 minute.

5. Make it soup: Increase the heat to medium-high, then add the cauliflower, the stock, salt, and nutmeg. Bring the soup to a boil, then reduce the heat to low. Cover the pot and simmer until the cauliflower is soft, about 20 minutes.

6. Puree the soup: Uncover and let the soup cool for 5 minutes. Blend the soup using an immersion blender (or transfer in batches to a blender or food processor).

continued on page 72

continued from page 71

7. Make the topping: Toast the sunflower seeds in a dry medium (9 or 10-inch) skillet over medium heat, stirring until fragrant and lightly golden, 3 to 4 minutes. Remove from the heat and stir in the cayenne.

8. Garnish and serve the soup: Pour the soup into 4 bowls and garnish with the sunflower seeds. Sprinkle the scallion greens on top and serve.

NUTRITIONAL INFORMATION (1 SERVING = 1½ CUPS SOUP, PLUS 2 TEASPOONS SEEDS) Calories 169, Total Fat 11.6 g 18%, Saturated Fat 1.4 g 7%, Trans Fat 0.0 g, Cholesterol 0.0 mg 0%, Sodium 572.6 mg 24%, Total Carb 14 g 5%, Dietary Fiber 4 g 16%, Sugars 2.7 g, Added Sugars 0 g, Protein 3.7 g 7%, Vitamin D 0.0 mcg 0%, Calcium 70.4 mg 7%, Iron 1.9 mg 11%, Potassium 326.6 mg 9%

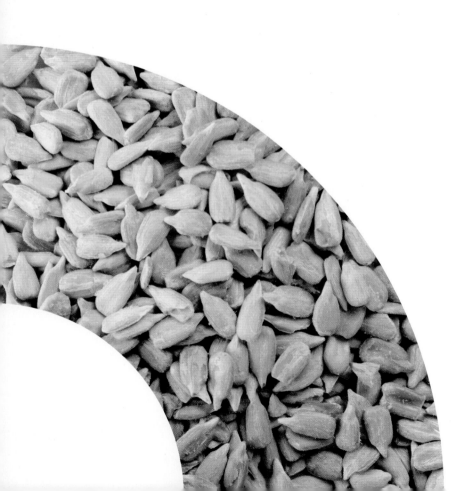

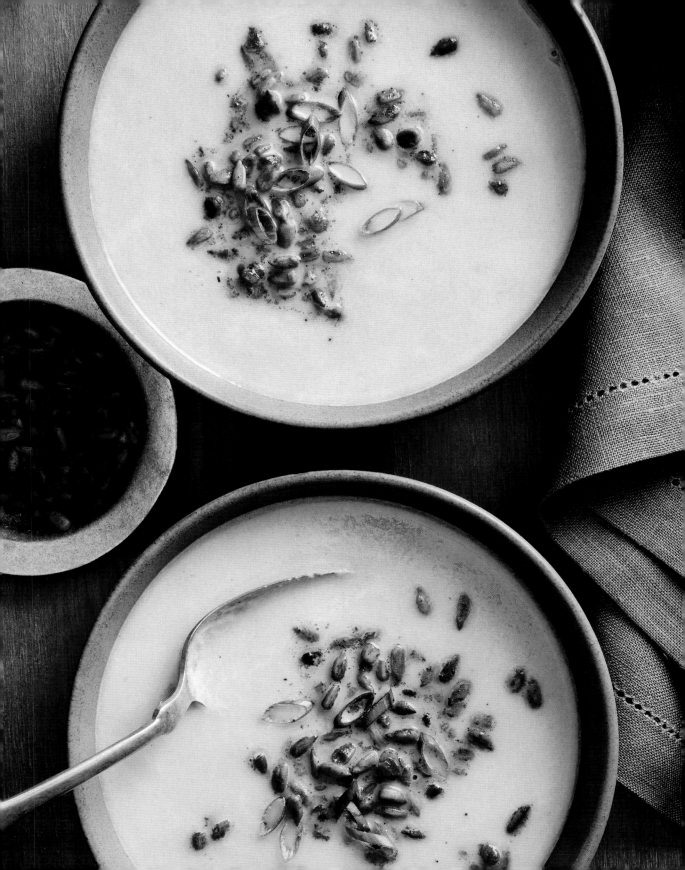

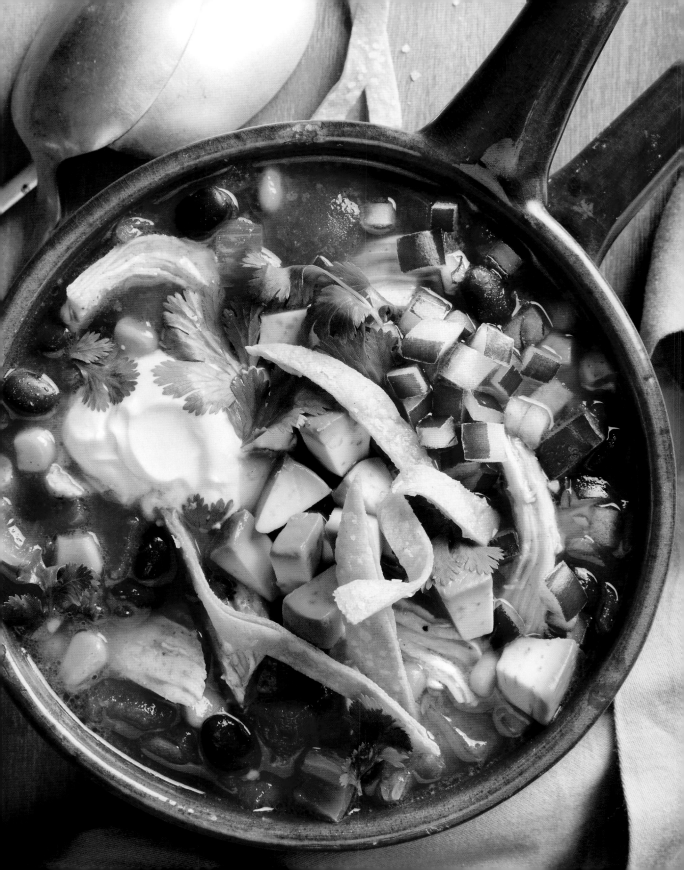

Creamy Tortilla Soup

1 tablespoon plus 2 teaspoons olive oil

1 small onion, diced

3 garlic cloves, minced

1½ teaspoons chili powder

1 teaspoon ground cumin

6 cups low-sodium chicken broth

2 14-ounce cans diced tomatoes (or 3 cups diced ripe tomatoes)

1 15-ounce can black beans, drained and rinsed

½ cup frozen corn kernels, thawed

2 teaspoons finely chopped chipotle chile in adobo sauce

¾ teaspoon kosher salt, plus more for seasoning

12 ounces cooked boneless, skinless chicken breast (such as from rotisserie chicken), shredded

4 6-inch corn tortillas

1 large avocado, halved, pitted, and diced

6 tablespoons finely diced red onion

6 tablespoons plain nonfat Greek yogurt

6 tablespoons chopped fresh cilantro

Tortilla soup is one of our favorite meals. There is something so satisfying about blending spicy chicken soup with chewy corn, crunchy tortilla strips, and creamy avocado. Using nonfat Greek yogurt lightens this soup up significantly without skimping on flavor.

SERVES 6   TOTAL TIME: 45 MINUTES

1. Sauté the vegetables and spices: Heat 1 tablespoon of the olive oil in a medium (at least 4-quart) pot over medium heat. Add the onion and cook, stirring, until lightly golden, 4 to 5 minutes. Add the garlic, chili powder, and cumin and cook, stirring, until the spices are fragrant, 1 to 2 minutes.

2. Make it soup: To the pot add the broth, tomatoes with their juices, black beans, corn, chipotle chile, and ½ teaspoon of the salt. Bring to a boil, reduce the heat to medium-low, and simmer uncovered until the broth thickens slightly and deepens in color, 20 to 30 minutes.

3. Bake the tortilla strips: While the soup is cooking, preheat the oven to 375°F.

4. Brush both sides of the tortillas with the remaining 2 teaspoons olive oil, then season with the remaining ¼ teaspoon salt. Stack the tortillas and use a sharp knife or a pizza cutter to cut them into ¼-inch-thick strips. Arrange the strips on a rimmed baking sheet and bake until crisp and lightly golden, about 15 minutes.

5. Finish and serve the soup: Stir the chicken into the soup and heat until warmed through, 3 to 4 minutes.

6. Taste the soup and season with additional salt, if necessary.

7. Divide the soup among 6 bowls. Top each bowl with a portion of the tortilla strips and a portion of the avocado cubes. Garnish each bowl with 1 tablespoon each of the red onion, yogurt, and cilantro.

NUTRITIONAL INFORMATION (1 SERVING = 1½ CUPS, PLUS ⅙ OF THE TORTILLA STRIPS AND ⅙ OF THE AVOCADO) Calories 393, Total Fat 13.8 g 21%, Saturated Fat 2.3 g 12%, Trans Fat 0.0 g, Cholesterol 50.2 mg 17%, Sodium 862.5 mg 36%, Total Carb 40.2 g 13%, Dietary Fiber 12.4 g 50%, Sugars 10.1 g, Added Sugars 0 g, Protein 31.8 g 64%, Vitamin D 2.8 mcg 1%, Calcium 149.4 mg 15%, Iron 4.4 mg 25%, Potassium 1124 mg 32%

Ruby Borscht

1 cup boiling water

1 ounce dried sliced shiitake mushrooms

2 tablespoons olive oil

1 large onion, diced

3 garlic cloves, minced

2½ cups thinly sliced green cabbage

2 medium carrots, finely diced

8 cups low-sodium vegetable broth

3 medium beets (about 1¼ pounds), peeled and cut into ¼-inch cubes

1 14-ounce can diced tomatoes

1 large waxy potato (12 ounces), peeled and cut into ¼-inch cubes

2 bay leaves

1 tablespoon white vinegar

2 teaspoons kosher salt, plus more for seasoning

1 teaspoon freshly ground black pepper

1 cup plain nonfat Greek yogurt

4 teaspoons finely chopped fresh dill

Lusciously ruby-red with soul-satisfying flavors, borscht is perfect for a chilly or blustery day. It's also full of delicious veggies in a variety of textures! Even though borscht itself is undeniably red, in Noom's world it's undoubtedly green.

SERVES 8 TOTAL TIME: 1 HOUR 15 MINUTES

1. Rehydrate the mushrooms: Put the boiling water in a small bowl and add the mushrooms. Soak until the mushrooms are soft, about 30 minutes.

2. Sauté the vegetables: While the mushrooms are soaking, heat the olive oil in a large (at least 6-quart) pot over medium heat. Add the onion and cook, stirring, until just tender, 5 to 6 minutes. Add the garlic and cook for 1 additional minute. Add the cabbage and carrots, and cook, stirring, until the vegetables begin to soften, 5 to 6 minutes.

3. Make it soup: Remove the mushrooms from the liquid with a slotted spoon and put them in another small bowl. Tip the soaking liquid into a third small bowl, leaving behind any sand or grit.

4. Pour the clean mushroom liquid into the pot along with the mushrooms, broth, beets, tomatoes with their juice, potato, and bay leaves.

5. Turn the heat to medium-high and bring to a boil. Reduce the heat to medium-low and simmer, partially covered, until the liquid thickens and darkens, about 1 hour. During the last 5 minutes of cooking, stir in the vinegar, 2 teaspoons salt, and the pepper.

6. Serve the soup: Remove the bay leaves, then divide the soup among 8 bowls. Serve each topped with 2 tablespoons of the yogurt and about ½ teaspoon of the dill.

NUTRITIONAL INFORMATION (1 SERVING = 1½ CUPS SOUP PLUS 2 TABLESPOONS YOGURT) Calories 163, Total Fat 3.9 g 6%, Saturated Fat 0.6 g 3%, Trans Fat 0.0 g, Cholesterol 1.4 mg 0%, Sodium 631.8 mg 26%, Total Carb 27.3 g 9%, Dietary Fiber 5.9 g 23%, Sugars 7.9 g, Added Sugars 0 g, Protein 6.5 g 13%, Vitamin D 5.5 mcg 1%, Calcium 129.4 mg 13%, Iron 2.8 mg 15%, Potassium 707.7 mg 20%

NOOM CHEF'S TIP: DRIED MUSHROOMS *Dried mushrooms are an alternative to fresh mushrooms, with a deeper, richer flavor, making them great for soups and sauces. They typically come in little packages at the supermarket. To use dried mushrooms, rinse them in a colander, and then soak them in hot water for about 30 minutes. Drain them, and then you can slice them or mince them and add them to your soup (or whatever needs that unique dried mushroom flavor).*

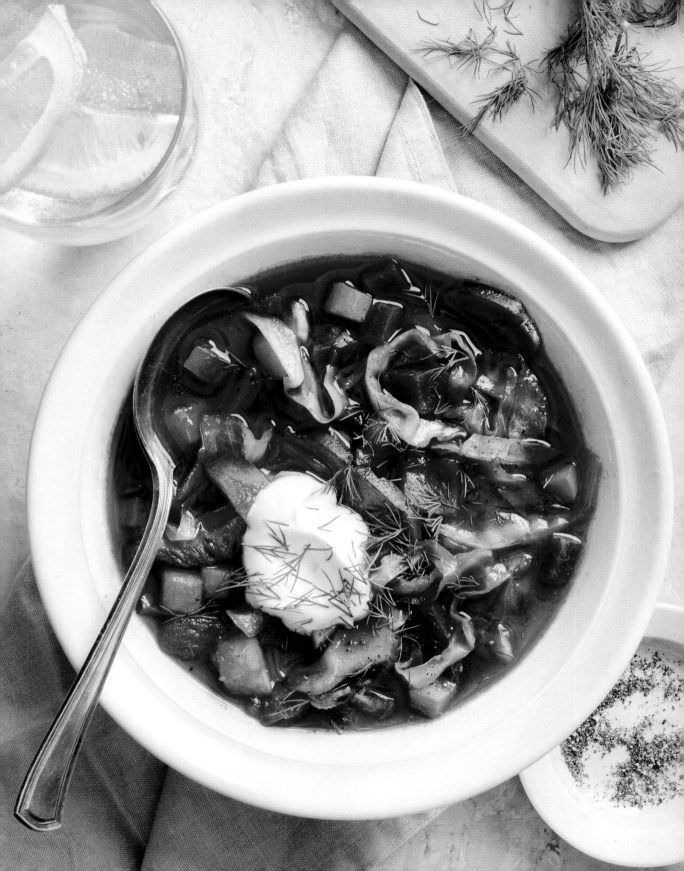

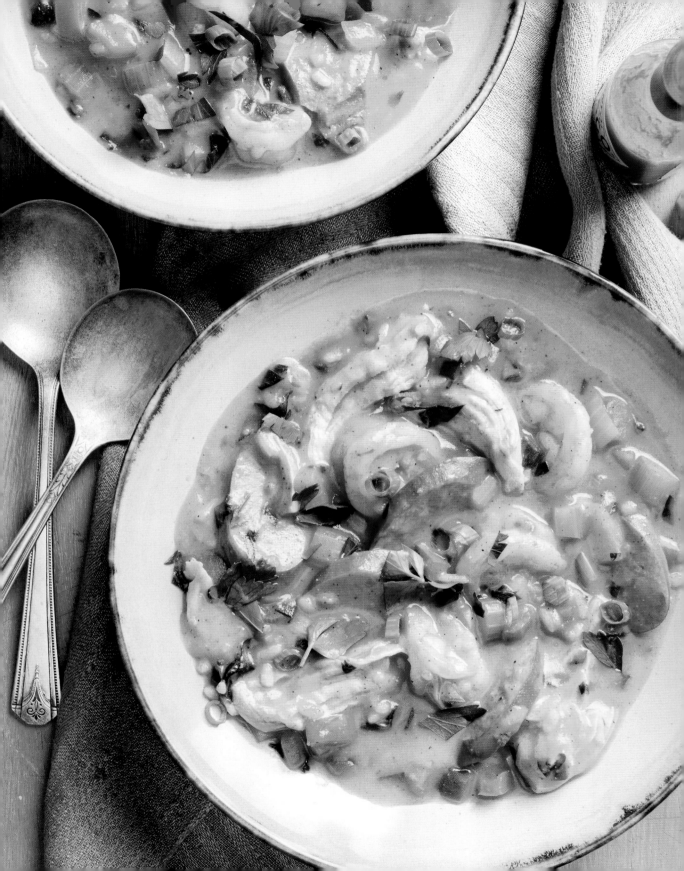

Shrimp & Chicken Gumbo

Gumbo is a classic thick Louisiana soup filled with seafood, sausage, chicken (or some combination of those), and lots of veggies in a rich liquid. This particular gumbo has some traditional elements, like filé powder (a thickener of powdered dried sassafras leaves). It skips other traditional ingredients, like okra (feel free to add, if you're a fan). If you're gluten free, you could substitute a gluten-free flour, such as brown rice or cassava flour, for the whole wheat flour.

½ cup white whole wheat flour (or whole wheat pastry flour)

1 cup nonfat milk

1 tablespoon olive oil

1 large onion, finely diced

6 celery stalks, finely diced

1 large green bell pepper, seeded, cored, and finely diced

4 ounces spicy chicken sausage, cut into thin rounds

5 garlic cloves, minced

2 tablespoons salt-free Cajun seasoning

1 teaspoon smoked paprika

1 teaspoon sweet paprika

6 cups low-sodium chicken broth

1 teaspoon kosher salt

12 ounces (or 14 ounces, if frozen) small (36–40 count) shrimp, thawed if frozen, cleaned, tails removed

2 cups (about 10 ounces) shredded cooked skinless white-meat chicken

2 tablespoons long-grain rice

1 tablespoon filé powder (optional)

½ cup chopped scallion greens

¼ cup chopped fresh parsley

Hot sauce, for serving (optional)

SERVES 8   TOTAL TIME: 1 HOUR

1. Make the roux: Place the flour in a medium (9- or 10-inch) dry skillet and cook over medium heat, frequently stirring and shaking the skillet so the flour covers the bottom of the pan in a thin layer, until the flour is golden and toasty, 4 to 5 minutes. Transfer to a bowl to cool for 5 minutes.

2. Whisk the milk into the flour until the flour is dissolved and there are no lumps.

3. Sauté the ingredients: Heat the olive oil in a large (at least 6-quart) heavy pot over medium heat. Add the onion, celery, pepper, and sausage and cook, stirring, until the onion is softened but not caramelized, 7 to 8 minutes.

4. Add the garlic, Cajun seasoning, and smoked and sweet paprikas and cook, stirring, 1 additional minute.

5. Make it soup: Add the broth and salt, bring to a boil over high heat, whisk in the roux, return to a boil, then reduce the heat to medium and continue cooking, stirring frequently, until the soup thickens, about 10 minutes.

6. Stir in the rice, return the soup to a boil, then reduce the heat to medium-low and simmer, stirring occasionally, until the liquid darkens and thickens, about 25 minutes.

7. Turn the heat up to medium-high and add the shrimp and chicken. Cook, stirring frequently, until the shrimp turns pink and the soup is heated through, 5 to 7 more minutes.

continued on page 80

continued from page 79

8. Serve the gumbo: Stir in the filé powder, if using. Stir in most of the scallion greens and most of the parsley, then divide the soup among 6 bowls. Garnish each with some of the remaining scallion greens and parsley. Serve with hot sauce, if desired.

NUTRITIONAL INFORMATION (1 SERVING = 1⅓ CUPS) Calories 218, Total Fat 5.5 g 8%, Saturated Fat 1.3 g 7%, Trans Fat 0.0 g, Cholesterol 88.8 mg 30%, Sodium 642.9 mg 27%, Total Carb 17.8 g 6%, Dietary Fiber 2.1 g 8%, Sugars 4.1 g, Added Sugars 0 g, Protein 24.6 g 49%, Vitamin D 17.1 mcg 4%, Calcium 143.9 mg 14%, Iron 2.1 mg 12%, Potassium 513.3 mg 15%

NOOM CHEF'S TIP: HOW TO MAKE A ROUX *Pronounced ROO, this soup starter is traditionally a combination of equal parts flour and fat. But we've broken with tradition to lighten up the roux. Our version is so easy that you might find you want to add a roux to all your soups!*

Just put about ½ cup flour in a small (8-inch) dry skillet over medium-high heat. Stir and shake the pan constantly until the flour turns golden brown. Be careful not to let it burn. When it's nicely tanned, remove it from the heat and whisk it into nonfat milk (or unsweetened nut, soy, or rice milk), then whisk that into your soup. As your soup simmers, it will thicken and get creamy and yummy. So easy, and much lighter than the butter bomb that is traditional roux.

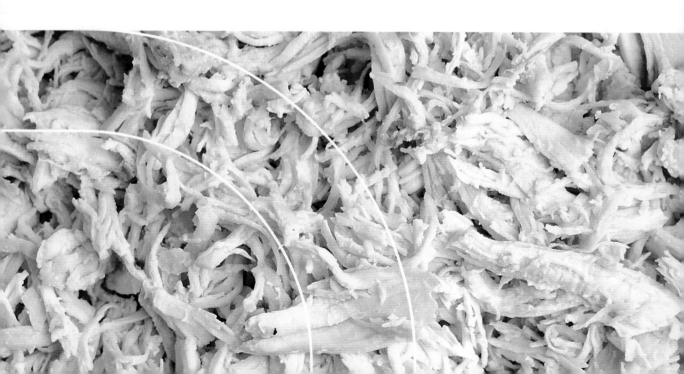

Spiced Chicken & Lentil Soup

Lentil soup is easy to make, and in this Indian-inspired version it's full of heady spices and tender chicken chunks. Use green or brown lentils here rather than red ones, which tend to fall apart in this preparation.

Before you cook your lentils, sift through them. Sometimes dried lentils have a little stone or two in the mix, and you aren't making stone soup!

SERVES 6 TOTAL TIME: 45 MINUTES

2 large boneless, skinless chicken breasts (about 2 pounds total)

Kosher salt and freshly ground black pepper

2 tablespoons olive oil

1 large onion, finely diced

1 tablespoon minced garlic

2 medium carrots, diced

2 celery stalks, diced

1 teaspoon garam masala

1¼ cups dried brown or green lentils, picked through and rinsed

6 cups chicken or vegetable broth (regular, not low sodium)

1 bay leaf

Chopped fresh parsley

1. Cook the chicken: Season the chicken generously with a little salt and black pepper.

2. Heat 1 tablespoon of the olive oil in a large (at least 6-quart) pot over medium heat. Add the chicken, cover the pot, and cook until evenly browned, 4 to 5 minutes per side, turning once. Lower the heat to medium-low and continue to cook until the chicken is no longer pink in the center, another 4 minutes.

3. Transfer the chicken to a plate to cool and pour off any pan juices.

4. Sauté the vegetables: Add the remaining tablespoon olive oil to the pot, then add the onion and cook over medium-low heat, stirring, until lightly golden, 8 to 9 minutes. Add the garlic and cook, stirring, 1 more minute. Add the carrots and celery, then season with ½ teaspoon salt. Cook, stirring, until vegetables are softened, about 5 minutes. Stir in the garam masala and cook briefly, stirring, until fragrant, about 1 minute.

5. Make it soup: Add the lentils to the pot, then pour in the broth. Add ½ teaspoon salt and the bay leaf. Bring to a boil over high heat, reduce the heat to medium, cover, and cook until the lentils are soft and just breaking apart, about 15 minutes.

continued on page 82

continued from page 81

6. Shred the chicken and add it to the pot. Lower the heat to medium-low and simmer until the chicken is warmed through and takes on some of the color of the soup, 9 to 10 minutes.

7. Serve the soup: Remove the bay leaf from the soup, then ladle the soup into 6 bowls. Garnish with the parsley and serve.

NUTRITIONAL INFORMATION (1 SERVING = 1⅔ CUPS) Calories 260, Total Fat 6.5 g 10%, Saturated Fat 1.0 g 5%, Trans Fat 0.0 g, Cholesterol 25.2 mg 8%, Sodium 1250.3 mg 52%, Total Carb 30 g 10%, Dietary Fiber 13.6 g 54%, Sugars 3.4 g, Added Sugars 0 g, Protein 20.6 g 41%, Vitamin D 2 mcg 0%, Calcium 57.9 mg 6%, Iron 3.8 mg 21%, Potassium 749.3 mg 21%

NOOM CHEF'S TIP *Garam masala is a popular spice blend used in Indian cooking. It typically contains a mix of ground cinnamon, pepper, coriander, cumin, and cardamom, although the different parts of India make their garam masala in various ways, so there is no one correct recipe. You can find garam masala in the spice aisle of your grocery store, or order it online. You could also substitute curry powder or use ground cumin with a dash each of cinnamon and black pepper.*

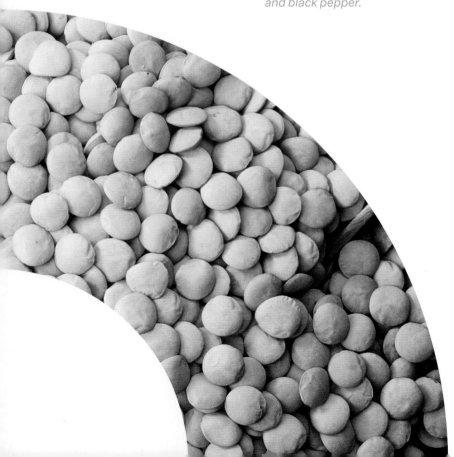

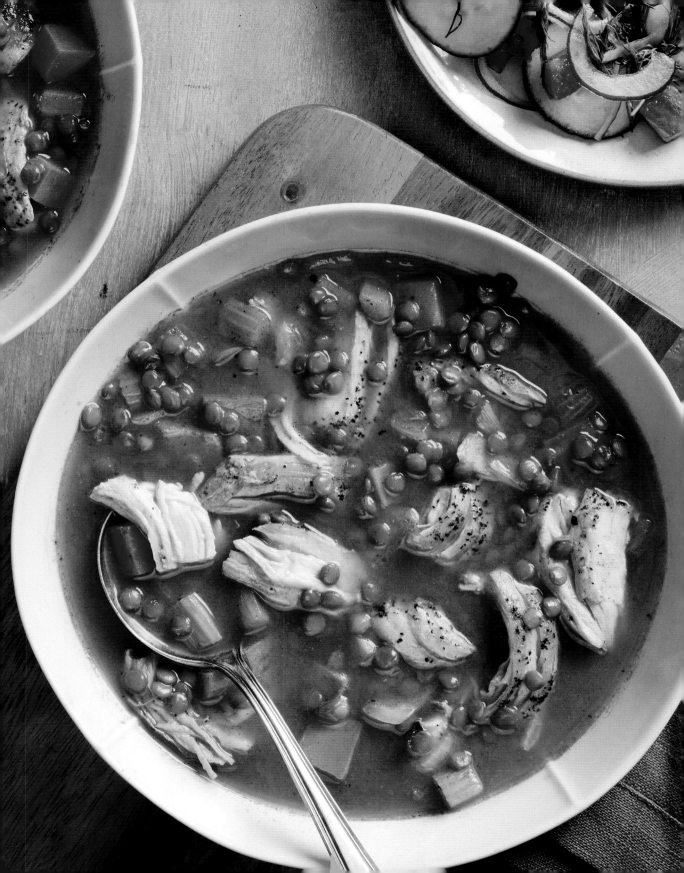

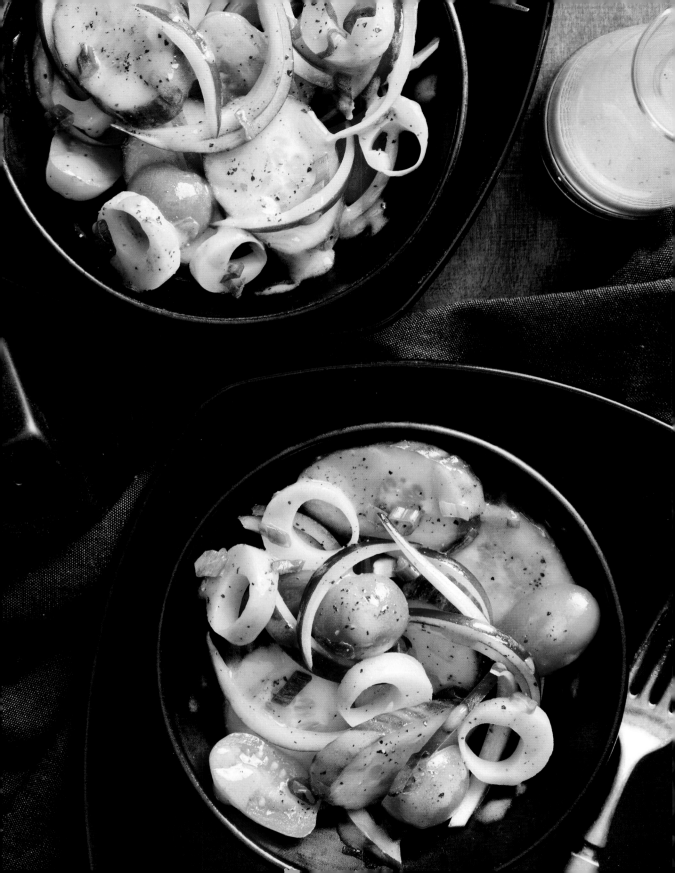

Cucumber & Hearts of Palm Salad

8 Persian or 2 large English cucumbers (about 1¼ pounds), trimmed and cut on the diagonal into ¼-inch slices

1 14-ounce can hearts of palm, drained, rinsed, and cut into ¼-inch slices

1 cup yellow or orange cherry tomatoes, halved

½ cup thinly sliced red onion

¼ cup thinly sliced scallion greens

Cucumber & Hearts of Palm Salad Dressing (page 110)

This light and refreshing salad combines adorable Persian cucumbers with hearts of palm, a tangy marinated vegetable with an almost meaty quality that can make a plain-Jane salad way more interesting. Brightly colored cherry tomatoes make it a party. This is great as a side dish, or toss in your favorite protein for a flavorful lunch!

SERVES 4   TOTAL TIME: 10 MINUTES

1. Assemble the salad: In a large bowl, combine the cucumbers, hearts of palm, tomatoes, red onion, and scallion greens.

2. Toss and serve the salad: Add the dressing to the salad and gently toss to incorporate. Season to taste with additional salt and pepper. Divide the salad among 4 bowls and serve.

NUTRITIONAL INFORMATION (1 SERVING = 1½ CUPS) Calories 155, Total Fat 7.7 g 12%, Saturated Fat 1.2 g 6%, Trans Fat 0.0 g, Cholesterol 0.0 mg 0%, Sodium 619.5 mg 26%, Total Carb 21.2 g 7%, Dietary Fiber 4.2 g 17%, Sugars 9 g, Added Sugars 0 g, Protein 4.6 g 9%, Vitamin D 0.0 mcg 0%, Calcium 99.7 mg 10%, Iron 4 mg 22%, Potassium 593.8 mg 17%

Surprise Chopped Salad with Creamy Dressing

If you've never tried making your own salad dressing, you're in for a serious treat. You can personalize homemade dressings however you like. This dressing is full of creamy lemony goodness—you can save it for other salads as well.

FOR THE SALAD

2 medium carrots, finely chopped

3 Persian cucumbers, finely chopped

2 cups finely chopped cauliflower florets

1 medium yellow bell pepper, finely chopped

1 medium red bell pepper, finely chopped

2 tablespoons thinly sliced scallion greens

FOR SERVING

Creamy Lemon Dressing (page 111)

2 tablespoons pomegranate seeds

2 tablespoons toasted pumpkin seeds

Salt and freshly ground black pepper

SERVES 4   TOTAL TIME: 15 MINUTES

1. Make the salad: In a large bowl, combine the carrots, cucumbers, cauliflower, yellow and red peppers, and scallion greens.

2. Serve the salad: Pour the dressing onto the salad and toss to incorporate. Sprinkle on the pomegranate and pumpkin seeds. Season to taste with salt and pepper. Divide the salad among 4 bowls and serve.

NUTRITIONAL INFORMATION (1 SERVING = 1½ CUPS) Calories 166, Total Fat 10.2 g 16%, Saturated Fat 1.7 g 8%, Trans Fat 0.0 g, Cholesterol 0.0 mg, Sodium 364.4 mg 15%, Total Carb 15.2 g 5%, Dietary Fiber 3.9 g 15%, Sugars 6.1 g, Added Sugars 0 g, Protein 5.5 g 11%, Vitamin D 0.0 mcg 0%, Calcium 51.2 mg 5%, Iron 1.5 mg 8%, Potassium 552.5 mg 16%

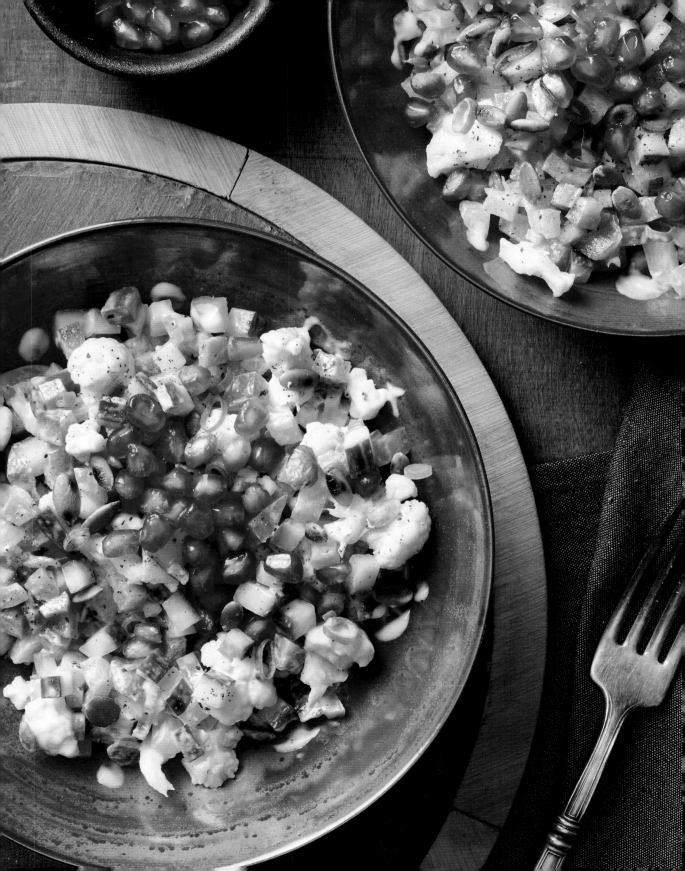

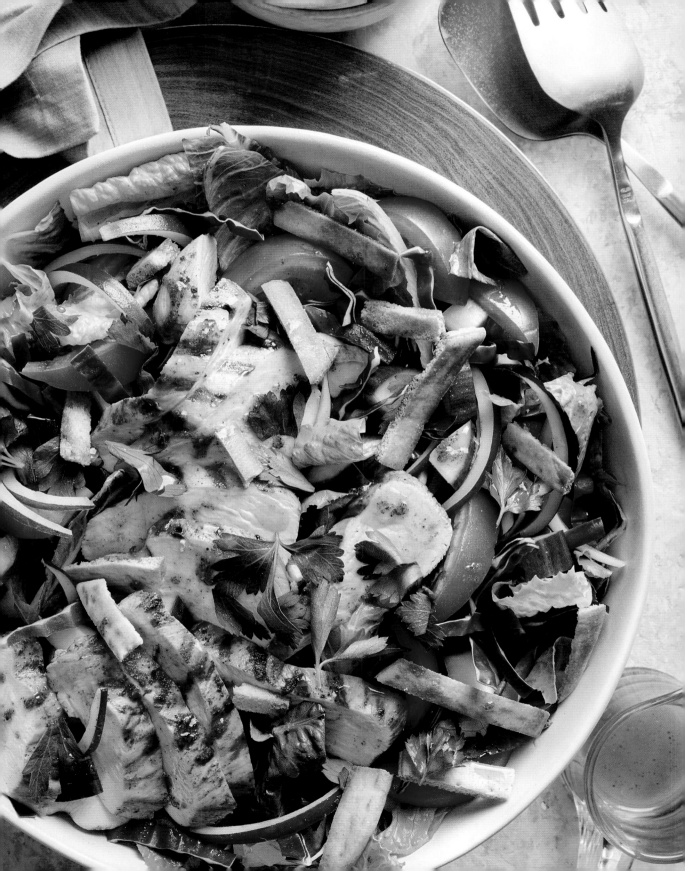

Grilled-Chicken Fattoush Salad

FOR THE CHICKEN

Zest of 1 lemon

1 tablespoon fresh lemon juice

1 tablespoon olive oil

3 garlic cloves, smashed

½ teaspoon ground sumac

½ teaspoon ground cumin

¼ teaspoon kosher salt

1 pound boneless, skinless chicken breasts

FOR THE PITA STRIPS

1 pita bread, split into 2 rounds

Olive oil cooking spray

¼ teaspoon kosher salt

FOR THE SALAD

2 heads romaine lettuce, chopped

3 vine-ripened medium tomatoes, cut into wedges

1 cup finely shredded red cabbage

4 Persian cucumbers, chopped

½ cup fresh parsley leaves, rinsed and dried

½ small red onion, thinly sliced

Fattoush Dressing (page 108)

Traditional fattoush salad is the Mediterranean equivalent of a Caesar salad, but with fried pita chunks instead of croutons and an olive-oil-based dressing instead of a creamy dressing. In our lighter version, the pita is cut into thin strips and toasted rather than fried, and the dressing is bursting with tangy lemon and sumac, which is one of our favorite spices (and not just because we love the deep red color).

SERVES 4 TOTAL TIME: 45 MINUTES

1. Marinate the chicken: Add the lemon zest and lemon juice to a medium bowl along with the olive oil, garlic, sumac, cumin, and salt. Add the chicken, toss to coat, and let it marinate on the counter while you prepare the pita.

2. Cut and bake the pita strips: Preheat the oven to 375°F.

3. Stack the pita halves, then halve them lengthwise with a serrated knife and cut them crosswise into ¼-inch strips. Arrange the strips on a rimmed baking sheet and spray the tops with the olive oil cooking spray for 3 seconds. Sprinkle with the salt and bake until the chips are crunchy and dry, about 12 minutes.

4. Grill the chicken: Heat a grill to medium-hot or preheat a stovetop grill pan over medium-high heat. Remove the chicken from the marinade, scrape off the garlic and lemon zest, and grill until the chicken has grill marks and is just cooked through, 2 to 3 minutes per side.

5. Transfer to a cutting board and cover with foil to keep warm.

6. Assemble and serve the salad: Arrange the lettuce, tomatoes, cabbage, cucumbers, parsley, and red onion on a serving platter. Slice the chicken into strips and scatter across the top. Scatter the pita strips over the chicken and drizzle with the dressing. Serve family style.

NUTRITIONAL INFORMATION (1 SERVING = 4 CUPS SALAD, WITH 4 OUNCES CHICKEN AND ¼ PITA) Calories 329, Total Fat 14.1 g 22%, Saturated Fat 2.2 g 11%, Trans Fat 0.0 g, Cholesterol 72.6 mg 24%, Sodium 515.1 mg 21%, Total Carb 23.5 g 8%, Dietary Fiber 5 g 20%, Sugars 7.2 g, Added Sugars 0 g, Protein 29 g 58%, Vitamin D 5.7 mcg 1%, Calcium 102.8 mg 10%, Iron 3 mg 17%, Potassium 1156.6 mg 33%

Lemony Cauliflower Tabbouleh

¼ cup sliced or chopped almonds

1 small head of cauliflower

1 large or 2 small bunches (about 4 ounces) fresh parsley

½ large bunch (about 1 ounce) fresh mint

4 firm, ripe medium red tomatoes, cored, seeded, and diced

8 scallions (white and green parts), trimmed and thinly sliced

2 tablespoons extra-virgin olive oil

Juice and zest of 1 lemon, plus more for serving

1 teaspoon kosher salt, plus more for serving

½ teaspoon ground cumin

Tabbouleh is a popular Middle Eastern salad made with bulgur wheat, parsley, and tomatoes. This lightened-up version uses cauliflower instead of bulgur wheat, which lends all the savory taste of the original with less caloric density. This tabbouleh is delicious on its own, heaped in a salad bowl, or served as a side dish.

SERVES 8   TOTAL TIME: 25 MINUTES

1. Roast the almonds: Preheat the oven to 350°F.

2. Arrange the almonds on a small baking sheet and roast until fragrant and lightly golden, 5 to 6 minutes.

3. Prepare the cauliflower: Grate the cauliflower on the large holes of a box grater into a large bowl, or pulse in a food processor until it resembles rice. You should have 1¾ to 2 cups.

4. Prepare the fresh herbs: Pick the leaves and tender stems from the parsley and mint, discarding the thicker stems.

5. Place the leaves in a large bowl, cover with very cold water, and swish them around for a few seconds. Remove the herbs from the water and dry them gently.

6. Working with a few handfuls of herbs at a time, chop the parsley and mint, making sure to move the herbs around while chopping them. (If you go over the herbs too many times in the same spot, they'll blacken.)

7. Assemble, dress, and toss the salad: Place the herbs in a large bowl. Add the cauliflower rice, then add the tomatoes and scallions. Drizzle on the olive oil and lemon juice, then sprinkle with 1 tablespoon of the lemon zest, 1 teaspoon salt, and the cumin. Toss well, then season to taste with more lemon zest and salt.

8. Serve the salad: Let the salad sit for 5 minutes, then serve immediately family style or place in 8 individual bowls. Garnish with the toasted almonds.

Note: This salad can be stored, covered, for up to 2 days in the fridge. Toss before serving to refresh the dressing.

NUTRITIONAL INFORMATION (1 SERVING = 1 CUP) Calories 78, Total Fat 5.2 g 8%, Saturated Fat 0.7 g 3%, Trans Fat 0.0 g, Cholesterol 0.0 mg 0%, Sodium 208.6 mg 9%, Total Carb 7.3 g 2%, Dietary Fiber 2.7 g 11%, Sugars 3.1 g, Added Sugars 0 g, Protein 2.6 g 5%, Vitamin D 0.0 mcg 0%, Calcium 52.9 mg 5%, Iron 1.5 mg 9%, Potassium 394.1 mg 11%

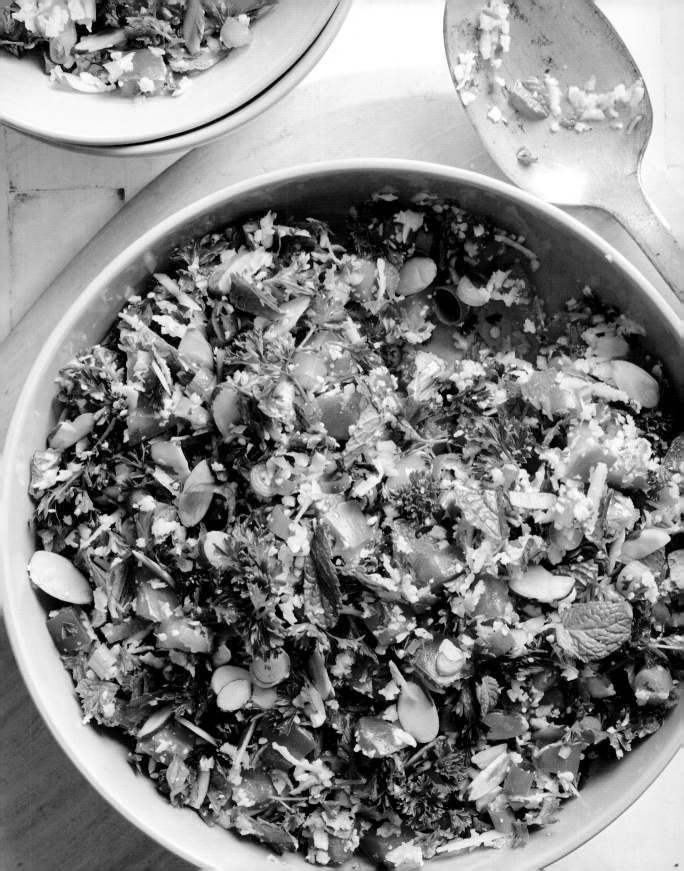

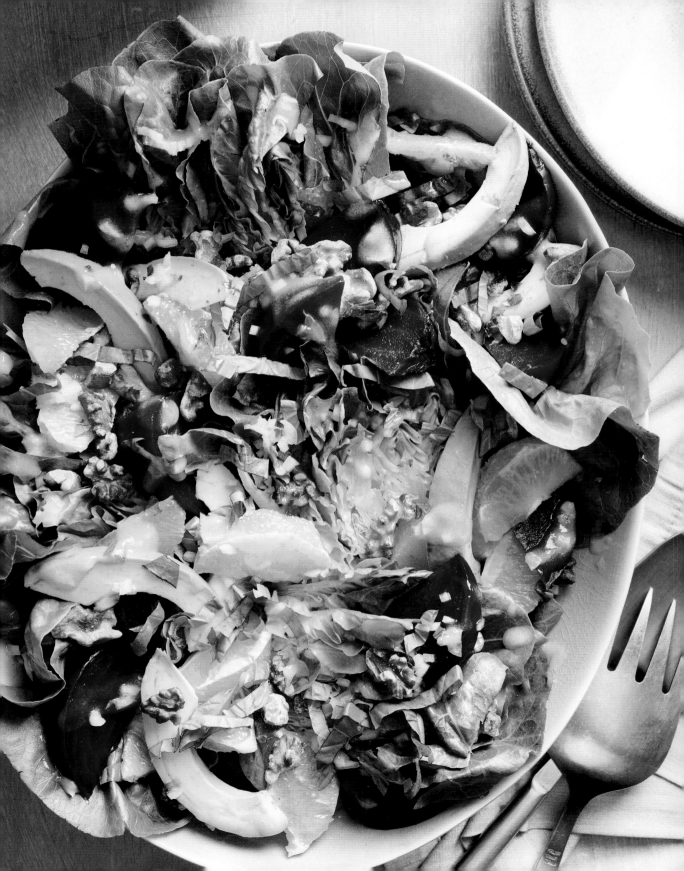

Little Gem Treasure Salad

Of all the many lettuces out there, Little Gem lettuce is probably the most charming (although of course this will be just as tasty with any of your favorite leafy greens). These cute little heads of romaine lettuce are only 4 to 6 inches high. Paired with jewel-toned beets, bright oranges, and crunchy walnuts, they make this salad like a little plate of treasure.

FOR THE WALNUTS, BEETS, AND ORANGES

¼ cup chopped walnuts

2 medium beets (about 1 pound), trimmed and scrubbed (see Note)

2 teaspoons olive oil

½ teaspoon kosher salt

3 medium oranges

FOR THE SALAD

4 heads of Little Gem lettuce, halved

½ small avocado, halved, pitted, and cut into thin wedges

Little Gem Treasure Salad Dressing (page 110)

¼ cup chopped fresh basil

SERVES 4 TOTAL TIME: 2 HOURS (INCLUDING ROASTING THE BEETS)

1. Roast the walnuts and beets: Preheat the oven to 400°F. Arrange the walnuts in a small baking dish.

2. Put the beets in the center of a 12-by-18-inch piece of aluminum foil. Drizzle each beet with 1 teaspoon olive oil and sprinkle each with ¼ teaspoon salt. Fold the foil over the beets to meet at the ends, then create a ½-inch fold and fold it over 2 more times to create a tight seal. Repeat with the 2 shorter ends to create a tight seal again.

3. Place the walnuts and the beet packet in the oven and roast until the walnuts are fragrant, 7 to 8 minutes. Remove the walnuts from the oven to cool.

4. Continue to roast the beets until they yield very slightly when pressed through the foil, another 1 to 1½ hours.

5. Remove the beet packet from the oven, cool for 1 hour, and then open the packet. Using your hands or a paper towel, slip the skins off the beets and discard. Cut the beets into wedges.

6. Section 2 of the oranges (see page 26 for photos and instructions), reserving any juices. Squeeze the third orange into a medium bowl and add the reserved juices; you should have about 3 tablespoons of juice.

7. Assemble the salad: Arrange the lettuce and beet wedges on a serving platter. Add the avocado and oranges. Drizzle with the dressing, then scatter on the toasted walnuts. Garnish the salad with the basil and serve family style.

Note: To save time, use 2 store-bought, vacuum-sealed cooked beets, cut into wedges. That will cut the total time down to 10 minutes.

NUTRITIONAL INFORMATION (1 SERVING = 3 CUPS) Calories 238, Total Fat 16.5 g 25%, Saturated Fat 2.1 g 10%, Trans Fat 0.0 g, Cholesterol 0.0 mg 0%, Sodium 438.9 mg 18%, Total Carb 21.7 g 7%, Dietary Fiber 7.3 g 29%, Sugars 13.4 g, Added Sugars 0 g, Protein 4.2 g 8%, Vitamin D 0.0 mcg 0%, Calcium 82.1 mg 8%, Iron 1.6 mg 9%, Potassium 651.8 mg 19%

Mediterranean Salad

When is a salad as filling as a meal? When you put chickpeas in it! Even though this is a side salad, it's perfect for a lighter main course because it's so full of protein and fiber. And if you enjoy a little heat with your meal, the satisfying spiciness from the jalapeños adds a lot of flavor.

Dijon Mustard Dressing (page 109)

6 vine-ripened small tomatoes (about 2 pounds), each cut into 8 wedges

1 cup canned chickpeas, drained and rinsed

½ cup thinly sliced red onion

1 ounce (about 4) sun-dried tomatoes (not oil-packed), thinly sliced

2 tablespoons capers, drained and rinsed

½ cup chopped fresh cilantro

SERVES 6   TOTAL TIME: 1 HOUR 15 MINUTES (INCLUDING MARINATING)

1. Assemble the salad: Add the dressing, tomatoes, chickpeas, red onion, sun-dried tomatoes, and capers to a bowl and gently toss to coat. Refrigerate to marinate for at least 1 hour and up to 24 hours.

2. Serve the salad: Toss the salad with the cilantro. Divide among 6 bowls and serve the salad chilled or at room temperature.

NUTRITIONAL INFORMATION (1 SERVING = 1 CUP) Calories 136, Total Fat 5.5 g 9%, Saturated Fat 0.8 g 4%, Trans Fat 0.0 g, Cholesterol 0.0 mg 0%, Sodium 436.6 mg 18%, Total Carb 19.4 g 6%, Dietary Fiber 4.7 g 19%, Sugars 6.5 g, Added Sugars 0 g, Protein 4.4 g 9%, Vitamin D 0.0 mcg 0%, Calcium 41.6 mg 4%, Iron 1.6 mg 9%, Potassium 608.4 mg 17%

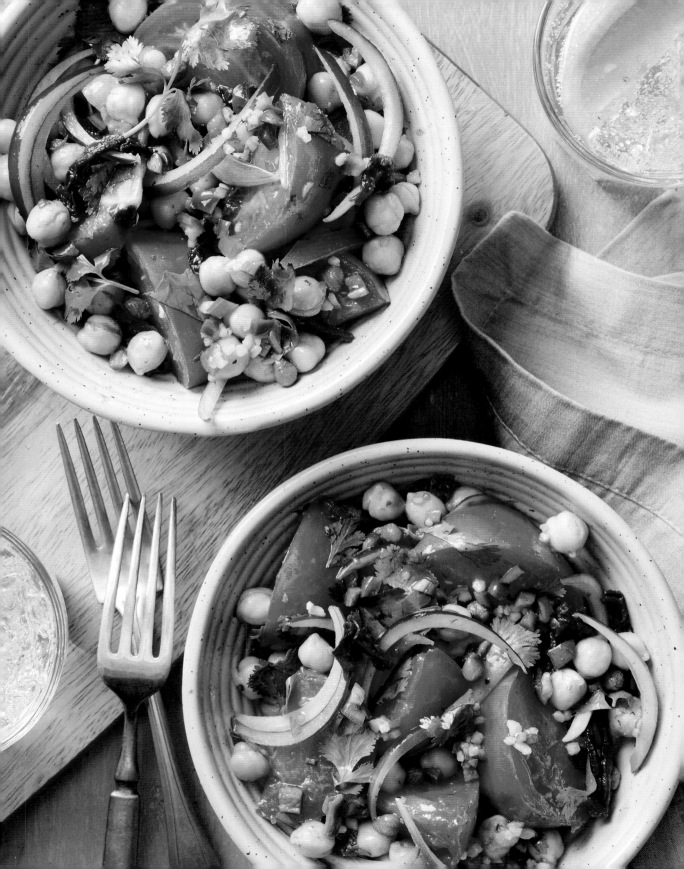

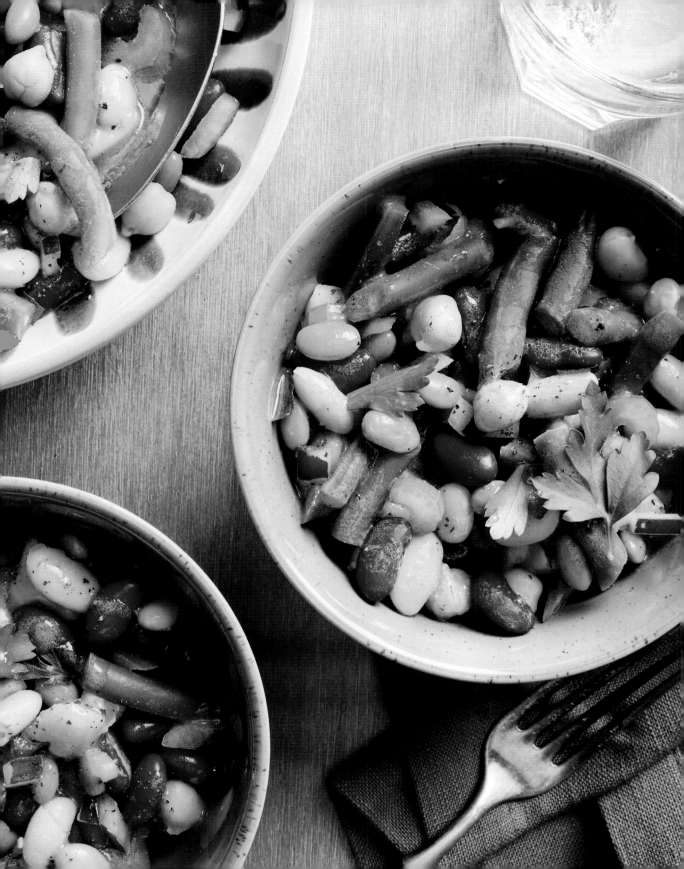

Tangy Five-Bean Salad

This quick and easy salad uses canned beans along with fresh green beans. It's full of protein and keeps well, making it a batch-cooking superstar. Enjoy it cold or at room temperature—and save those leftovers, because this salad tastes even better the next day.

SERVES 8   TOTAL TIME: 15 MINUTES

FOR THE SALAD

Kosher salt

8 ounces fresh green beans, trimmed and cut into 1½-inch pieces

2 cups ice cubes

1 15-ounce can chickpeas, drained and rinsed

1 15-ounce can cannellini beans, drained and rinsed

1 15-ounce can kidney beans, drained and rinsed

1¼ cups frozen edamame, thawed

3 celery stalks, thinly sliced

½ small red onion, finely chopped

¼ cup chopped fresh parsley

Tangy Five-Bean Salad Dressing (page 110)

1. Cook the green beans: Bring a medium (at least 4-quart) pot of generously salted water to a boil. Add the green beans and cook until tender-crisp, 3 to 4 minutes.

2. While the beans are cooking, fill a medium bowl halfway with cold water and add the ice cubes. Drain the beans in a colander, then transfer them to the ice water bath and cool for 1 to 2 minutes. Drain again.

3. Assemble the salad: Add the green beans to a large bowl. Add the chickpeas, cannellini beans, kidney beans, edamame, celery, red onion, and parsley, and stir to combine.

4. Toss and serve the salad: Add the dressing to the salad and toss to combine. Season to taste with additional salt and pepper. Transfer the bean salad to a serving bowl, or portion into 6 individual bowls. Serve at room temperature, or chill first, if desired.

NUTRITIONAL INFORMATION (1 SERVING = 1 CUP) Calories 228, Total Fat 5.5 g 8%, Saturated Fat 0.7 g 3%, Trans Fat 0.0 g, Cholesterol 0.0 mg 0%, Sodium 682.7 mg 28%, Total Carb 35.9 g 12%, Dietary Fiber 9.6 g 38%, Sugars 5.8 g, Added Sugars 0 g, Protein 10.9 g 22%, Vitamin D 0.0 mcg 0%, Calcium 90.2 mg 9%, Iron 2.8 mg 15%, Potassium 529.8 mg 15%

NOOM CHEF'S TIP *Legumes have that satisfyingly dense texture that can stand in for meat, but they also complement meaty dishes (hello, chili) and can help you eat a little less meat while still getting plenty of protein and satisfaction from each meal. On top of all those stellar benefits, legumes contain a lot of B vitamins, iron, calcium, and zinc. They are great in salads, make a mean veggie burger, and (dare we say?) are even better in soups. Wow, legumes, is there anything you can't do?*

B.L.A.T. Salad with Ranch Dressing

FOR THE BACON AND CRUMBS

4 ounces turkey bacon (about 3 slices, depending on thickness)

¼ cup panko or other bread crumbs

Olive oil cooking spray

¼ teaspoon kosher salt

FOR THE SALAD

1 large head iceberg lettuce, chopped

2 ripe beefsteak tomatoes, cut into chunks

1 small avocado, halved, pitted, and diced

½ cup thinly sliced red onion

Best-Ever Ranch Dressing (page 109)

If you haven't made your own ranch dressing yet, what are you waiting for? Homemade ranch dressing is so easy and so good that you'll wonder why you ever bought it in a bottle, and we bet our Best-Ever Ranch Dressing really will be the best you've ever tried. When you use it to dress juicy iceberg lettuce and tomatoes, savory low-fat turkey bacon, creamy avocado, and a sprinkle of crunchy panko, you'll get all the great flavors of a BLT sandwich.

SERVES 6 TOTAL TIME: 30 MINUTES

1. Cook the bacon and toast the crumbs: Arrange 2 racks in the bottom and top third of the oven. Preheat the oven to 400°F.

2. Arrange the bacon on a parchment-lined rimmed baking sheet.

3. Spread out the panko in a single layer in a small baking dish and spray for 3 seconds with the olive oil cooking spray. Sprinkle with the salt.

4. Place the crumbs on the bottom rack and the bacon on the top rack of your oven. Bake the crumbs until golden and toasty, 5 to 6 minutes, then remove from the oven to cool.

5. Continue to cook the turkey bacon until the top side is sizzling, another 4 minutes or so, then flip the bacon strips and cook until the underside is crisp and sizzling, another 6 to 7 minutes. Cool and break the bacon into pieces.

6. Assemble the salad and serve: Arrange the lettuce in a large salad bowl. Scatter the bacon over the lettuce, then add the tomatoes, avocado, and red onion. Drizzle Best-Ever Ranch Dressing over all, and sprinkle the salad with the toasted bread crumbs. Serve family style.

NUTRITIONAL INFORMATION (1 SERVING = 3 CUPS) Calories 150, Total Fat 8.3 g 13%, Saturated Fat 1.9 g 10%, Trans Fat 0.1 g, Cholesterol 20.3 mg 7%, Sodium 463.5 mg 19%, Total Carb 13 g 4%, Dietary Fiber 4.2 g 17%, Sugars 7 g, Added Sugars 0 g, Protein 8.2 g 16%, Vitamin D 10.6 mcg 3%, Calcium 90.8 mg 9%, Iron 1.3 mg 7%, Potassium 545.4 mg 16%

NOOM CHEF'S TIP: DIY BUTTERMILK *When you need buttermilk for a recipe but don't have any on hand, you can make a respectable substitute in a few minutes. To make 1 cup of buttermilk substitute, measure 1 tablespoon white vinegar or lemon juice into a measuring cup. Fill the cup with any kind of milk (nonfat, low-fat, whole, or plant-based) and let it sit for about 10 minutes. You can then whisk it into your recipe.*

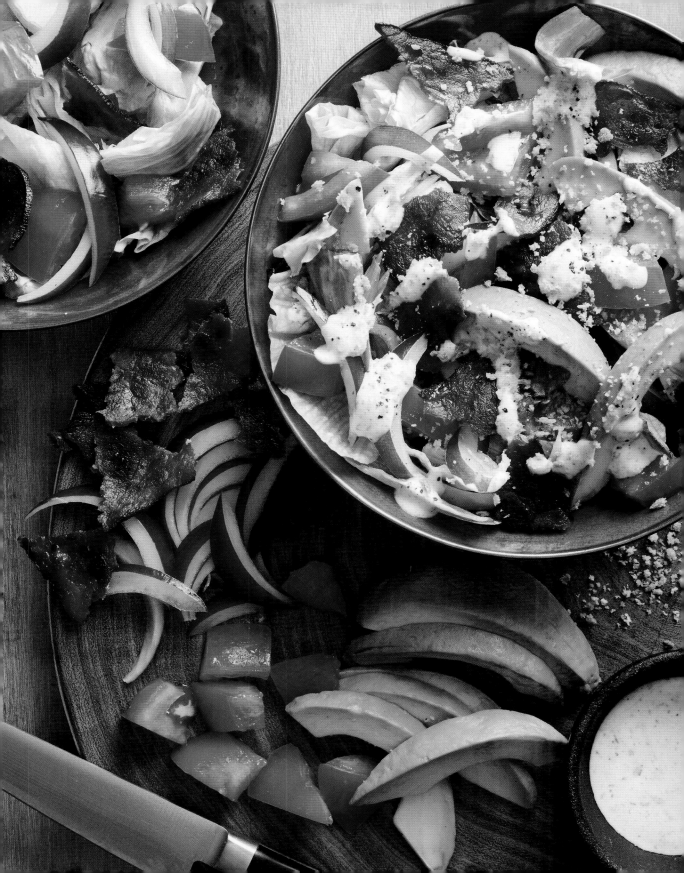

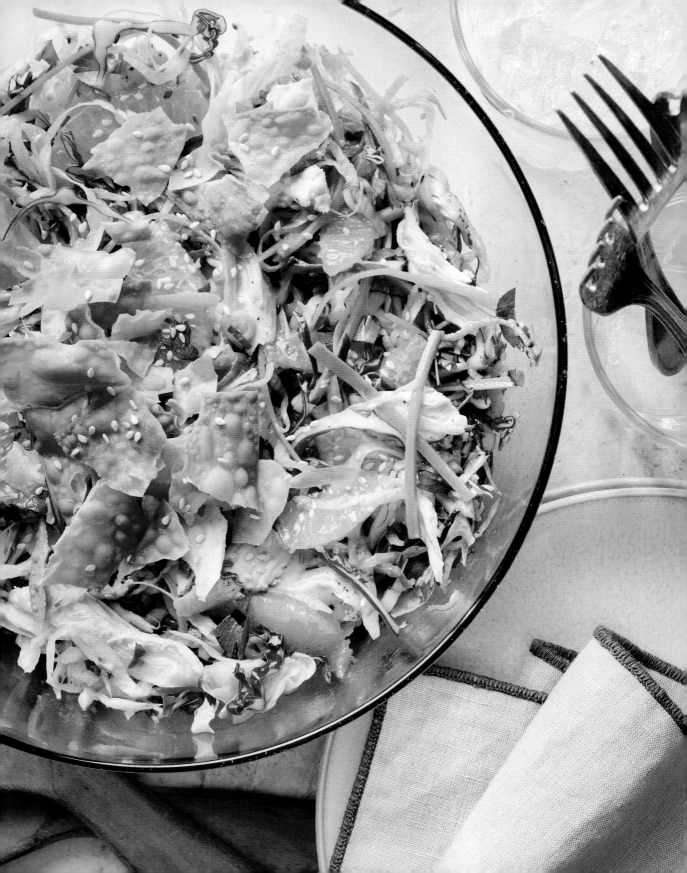

Chinese Chicken Salad

This satisfying salad is studded with juicy oranges and full of crunch from the cabbage and fried wanton strips. The sesame dressing is so good that you may want to make a double batch for use on future salads—it will keep well in a covered jar or bottle on the counter for about 4 days. Just shake it up and drizzle it on everything.

SERVES 4   TOTAL TIME: 30 MINUTES

FOR THE WONTONS

4 wonton wrappers

1 teaspoon canola or other light vegetable oil

¼ teaspoon kosher salt

FOR THE SALAD

2 medium (1 pound) cooked store-bought boneless, skinless white-meat chicken breasts (such as from a rotisserie chicken), shredded (or buy pre-shredded)

1 large head iceberg lettuce, very thinly sliced

2 cups thinly shredded red cabbage

¾ cup roughly chopped fresh cilantro leaves or Italian flat parsley leaves

2 large carrots, cut into thin julienne strips

3 scallions (green and white parts), thinly sliced

Chinese Chicken Salad Dressing (page 108)

1 orange, segmented, plus any accumulated juice

2 tablespoons sesame seeds, toasted

1. Make the wontons: Preheat the oven to 350°F.

2. Arrange the wontons on a baking sheet, brush with the oil, season with the salt, and bake until crisp and golden, 10 to 12 minutes.

3. Make the salad and serve: Place the chicken in a large bowl. Add the lettuce, red cabbage, cilantro, carrots, and scallions. Pour in the dressing. Add the orange segments and any orange juice, then gently toss to coat.

4. Use your hands to crush the wonton wrappers into bite-sized pieces and add them to the bowl. Sprinkle in the sesame seeds and divide among 4 salad bowls.

NUTRITIONAL INFORMATION (1 SERVING = 4 CUPS) Calories 485, Total Fat 23.9 g 37%, Saturated Fat 3.7 g 18%, Trans Fat 0.0 g, Cholesterol 98.7 mg 33%, Sodium 1850.8 mg 77%, Total Carb 33.3 g 11%, Dietary Fiber 5.4 g 22%, Sugars 20.1 g, Added Sugars 0 g, Protein 37 g 74%, Vitamin D 0.0 mcg 0%, Calcium 104.9 mg 10%, Iron 2.4 mg 13%, Potassium 843.4 mg 24%

Lemon, Pepper & Parm Chicken Salad

The advantage of chicken cutlets, or thinly sliced chicken breast, is that they cook quickly, as well as helping you stretch a large chicken breast for use in multiple meals. Sometimes you can find packaged chicken cutlets in the store or ask the butcher to prepare them, but you can also make your own (see page 29). If you want to grate and shave the Parmigiano-Reggiano cheese yourself, you can use a microplane for grating and a vegetable peeler for shaving. The total amount you'll need is approximately 1 ounce.

Lemon, Pepper & Parm Chicken Salad Dressing (page 108)

4 4-ounce chicken cutlets

4 cups arugula

1 cup cherry tomatoes, halved

¼ cup thinly sliced red onion

2 tablespoons shaved Parmigiano-Reggiano cheese

Kosher salt and freshly ground black pepper

SERVES 4   TOTAL TIME: 25 MINUTES

1. Grill the chicken: Heat a grill to very hot or preheat a stovetop grill pan over high heat.

2. Measure about ¼ cup of the dressing into a small bowl and brush it all over the chicken. Grill the chicken until grill marks form and it's just cooked through, 2 to 3 minutes per side.

3. Assemble the salad and serve: In a large bowl, combine the arugula, tomatoes, and onion. Add the remaining dressing and gently toss.

4. Arrange a piece of grilled chicken on each plate and top each with about 1⅔ cups of the salad mixture. Sprinkle equal amounts of the shaved cheese on each plate. Season to taste with salt and pepper, then serve.

NUTRITIONAL INFORMATION (1 SERVING = 1½ CUPS SALAD, WITH 1 CHICKEN CUTLET)
Calories 303, Total Fat 16.1 g 25%, Saturated Fat 3.7 g 18%, Trans Fat 0.1 g, Cholesterol 80.4 mg 27%, Sodium 518.8 mg 22%, Total Carb 8.6 g 3%, Dietary Fiber 1.8 g 7%, Sugars 3.1 g, Added Sugars 0 g, Protein 31 g 62%, Vitamin D 5.7 mcg 1%, Calcium 180.6 mg 18%, Iron 1.7 mg 9%, Potassium 681.9 mg 19%

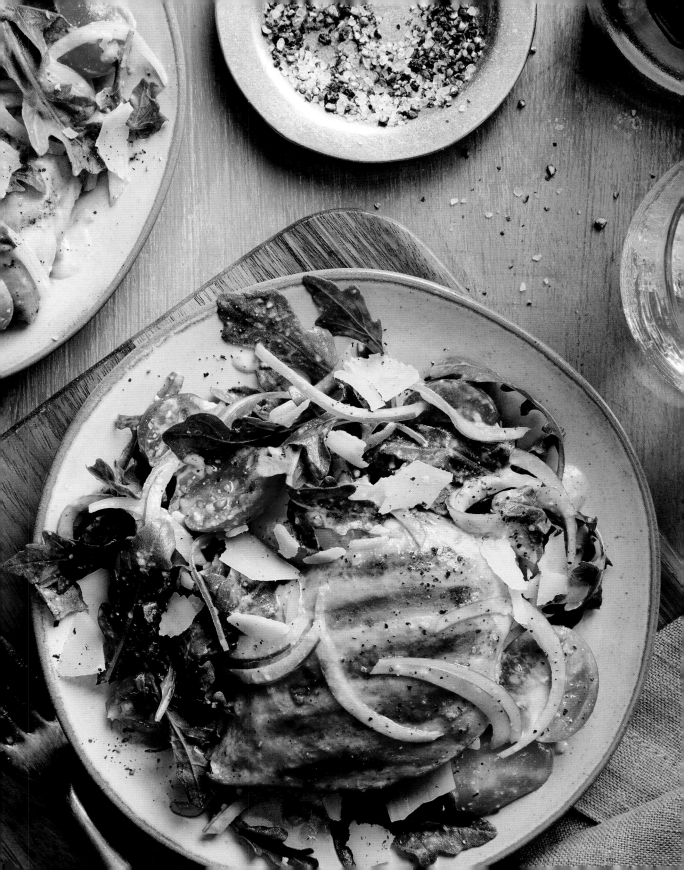

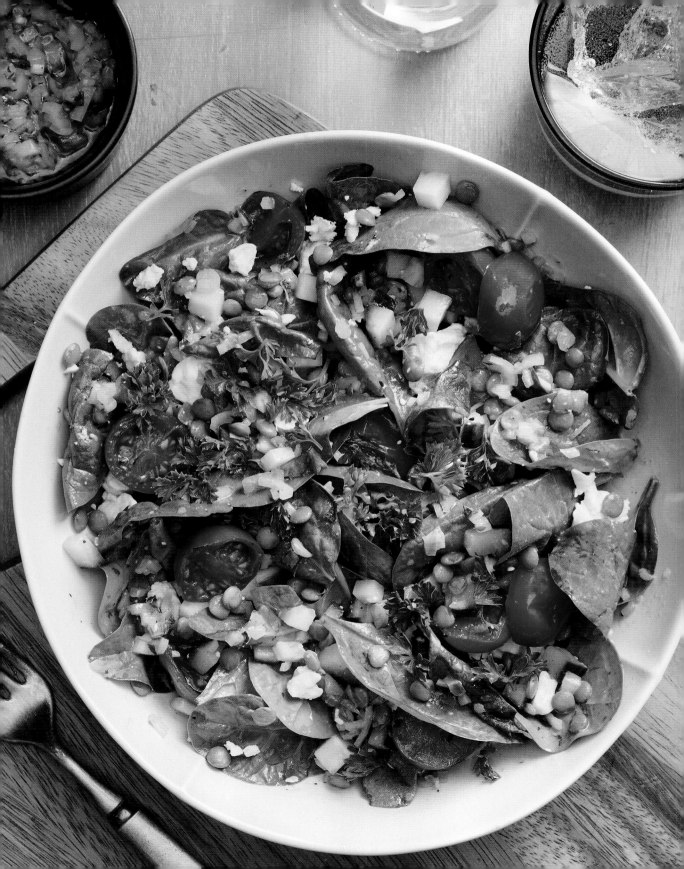

Lentils & Greens with Roasted Tomatoes

Lentils give this filling salad a meaty and satisfying texture, as well as a boost of protein without meat. Use any kind of lentils except red, which get too mushy when cooked. To save time, you could also use 2 cups drained and rinsed canned lentils.

FOR THE LENTILS

2 teaspoons kosher salt

1¼ cups dried green or brown lentils, rinsed and drained

1 garlic clove, smashed

1 teaspoon ground cumin

1 bay leaf

FOR THE TOMATOES

2 cups cherry tomatoes, halved

1 tablespoon olive oil

¾ teaspoon Kosher salt

FOR THE SALAD

2 cups lightly packed baby spinach leaves, stems trimmed

3 Persian cucumbers, trimmed, quartered lengthwise, and cut into ¼-inch pieces

½ cup crumbled feta

Dijon Mustard Dressing (page 109)

Salt and freshly ground black pepper

¼ cup chopped fresh parsley

SERVES 6   TOTAL TIME: 1 HOUR 15 MINUTES

1. Preheat the oven to 400°F.

2. Make the lentils: Fill a medium saucepan two-thirds full with water. Add the salt, lentils, garlic, cumin, and bay leaf. Bring to a boil, then reduce the heat to low and cook, stirring occasionally, until lentils are just past al dente (taste at around 18 minutes to check), 20 to 22 minutes.

3. Drain and cool the lentils, then discard the bay leaf and garlic clove.

4. Make the tomatoes: Arrange the tomatoes on a rimmed baking sheet, drizzle with the olive oil and sprinkle with the salt, and roast until some of the tomatoes burst and the rest are charred or shriveled, about 20 minutes. Remove from the oven to cool.

5. Assemble the salad and serve: In a large bowl, combine the lentils and roasted tomatoes, then add the spinach, cucumbers, and feta. Toss gently to combine. Pour the dressing over the salad and toss to coat. Season with the salt and pepper to taste and garnish with the parsley. Divide the salad among 4 salad bowls and serve warm, at room temperature, or chilled.

Note: This salad keeps for 1 day covered in the refrigerator.

NUTRITIONAL INFORMATION (1 SERVING = 1½ CUPS) Calories 301, Total Fat 14.6 g 23%, Saturated Fat 3.5 g 18%, Trans Fat 0.0 g, Cholesterol 11.1 mg 4%, Sodium 689.5 mg 29%, Total Carb 30.3 g 10%, Dietary Fiber 13.8 g 55%, Sugars 3.9 g, Added Sugars 0 g, Protein 13.4 g 27%, Vitamin D 2 mcg 0%, Calcium 121.9 mg 12%, Iron 4.2 mg 23%, Potassium 675.2 mg 19%

NOOM CHEF'S TIP: CUCUMBER SIZING *We love crunchy, juicy cucumbers, but sometimes cucumbers can have a bitter taste, too many seeds, or a tough skin. That's why we love Persian cucumbers—those little cucumbers that come grouped in packages. They have a soft skin, sweet flavor, and very few small seeds, so you don't have to peel or seed them. They are sometimes called baby cucumbers or mini cucumbers.*

Veggie-Packed Summer Deli Pasta Salad

You can make this recipe with any shape of stubby pasta, or even orzo or spaghetti if you want to live on the edge. Skim the pasta out of the hot water with a handheld strainer or skimmer for this recipe because you'll need to use the boiling water to cook the broccolini.

FOR THE PASTA AND VEGGIE

Kosher salt

8 ounces whole-grain fusilli or penne pasta

1 10-ounce bunch broccolini, baby broccoli, or broccoli rabe (florets and leaves), tough stems trimmed and discarded

FOR THE SALAD

1 cup cherry tomatoes, halved

1 cup thinly sliced red onion

6 ounces sliced smoked turkey breast, cut into ½-inch strips

3 ounces mini mozzarella balls (or a 3-ounce piece of fresh mozzarella, cut into ½-inch cubes)

1 ounce thinly sliced salami, cut into matchsticks

½ cup pitted green olives, any type (fancier ones, such as Castelvetrano, may need to be hand-pitted), sliced

¼ pepperoncini, drained and chopped

¼ cup grated supermarket-style Parmesan cheese

Kosher salt and freshly ground black pepper

Veggie-Packed Summer Deli Pasta Salad Dressing (page 109)

SERVES 10 TOTAL TIME: 35 MINUTES

1. Boil the pasta: Fill a large (at least 6-quart) pot with water and generously salt (about 1 teaspoon salt per quart). Add the pasta and cook according to package directions until al dente. Use a spider strainer or skimmer to transfer the pasta from the water to a colander, then rinse in cold water to stop the cooking. Drain and set the pasta aside. Leave the cooking water in the pot.

2. Boil the broccolini: Return the pasta water to a boil and gently lower the broccolini into the pot using the spider strainer or skimmer. Cook until the broccolini turns bright green, about 2 minutes.

3. Drain, then run cold water over the broccolini to stop the cooking and maintain the bright green color. Drain, pat dry very well, then chop the broccolini into 1-inch lengths.

4. Assemble and serve the salad: Place the pasta and broccolini in a large serving bowl. Stir in the tomatoes, red onion, turkey strips, mozzarella balls, salami sticks, olives, pepperoncini, and Parmesan. Toss to combine, then season to taste with salt and pepper. Serve the pasta salad family style, or portion into individual bowls with the dressing on the side.

Note: The salad can be kept in a covered container for up to 5 days.

NUTRITIONAL INFORMATION (1 SERVING = 1 CUP) Calories 209, Total Fat 10.3 g 16%, Saturated Fat 2.7 g 14%, Trans Fat 0.1 g, Cholesterol 19.2 mg 6%, Sodium 477.4 mg 20%, Total Carb 20.6 g 7%, Dietary Fiber 4 g 16%, Sugars 1.7 g, Added Sugars 0 g, Protein 11.2 g 22%, Vitamin D 1.9 mcg 0%, Calcium 82.4 mg 8%, Iron 2.2 mg 12%, Potassium 144.6 mg 4%

NOOM CHEF'S TIP: BROCCOLI 101 *Broccolini, baby broccoli, broccoli rabe—what's the difference? Broccolini is a hybrid of regular broccoli and Chinese broccoli, with longer, more slender stems and tender flowers. Baby broccoli is simply regular broccoli before it's all grown up, so it's more tender and sweeter. Broccoli rabe isn't actually related to broccoli—it's also called rapini.*

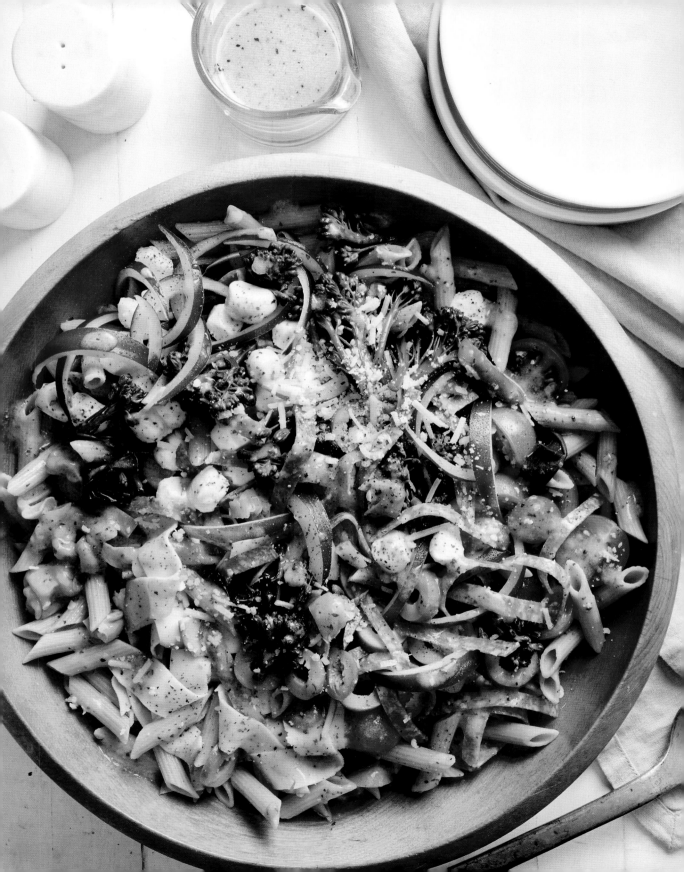

Irresistible Homemade Dressings

Fattoush Dressing

2 tablespoons fresh lemon juice

2 tablespoons olive oil

½ teaspoon ground sumac

¼ teaspoon kosher salt

¼ teaspoon freshly ground black pepper

Combine the lemon juice with the olive oil, sumac, salt, and black pepper in a small jar. Shake until creamy, then chill until ready to use.

Chinese Chicken Salad Dressing

2 garlic cloves

⅓ cup rice vinegar

¼ cup olive oil

3 tablespoons water

2 tablespoons Dijon mustard

1½ tablespoons soy sauce

3 teaspoons pure maple syrup

2 teaspoons toasted sesame oil

1 teaspoon sriracha sauce

Add the garlic, vinegar, olive oil, water, mustard, soy sauce, maple syrup, sesame oil, and sriracha to a blender and blend until smooth, about 30 seconds.

Lemon, Pepper & Parm Chicken Salad Dressing

2 tablespoons finely grated Parmigiano-Reggiano cheese

4 garlic cloves

¼ cup fresh lemon juice

2 tablespoons olive oil

2 tablespoons tahini

2 tablespoons plain nonfat Greek yogurt

1 tablespoon Dijon mustard

1 anchovy fillet (or ½ teaspoon fish sauce)

1 teaspoon Worcestershire sauce, or more as desired

½ teaspoon kosher salt

¼ teaspoon freshly ground black pepper

In a blender, combine the grated cheese, garlic, lemon juice, olive oil, tahini, yogurt, and mustard. Add the anchovy, then the Worcestershire sauce, salt, and pepper to the blender and blend until smooth.

Dijon Mustard Dressing

2 tablespoons minced shallot

¼ cup olive oil

3 tablespoons red wine vinegar

2 teaspoons Dijon mustard

1 tablespoon chopped fresh oregano

¼ teaspoon kosher salt

½ teaspoon freshly ground black pepper

In a small jar with a tight-fitting lid, combine the shallot, olive oil, vinegar, mustard, oregano, salt, and pepper, and shake until emulsified.

Veggie-Packed Summer Deli Pasta Salad Dressing

¼ cup red wine vinegar

¼ cup olive oil

2 teaspoons Dijon mustard

1 teaspoon dried oregano

1 teaspoon dried basil

½ teaspoon kosher salt

Combine the vinegar, olive oil, mustard, oregano, basil, and salt in a large bowl, and whisk to combine.

Best-Ever Ranch Dressing

½ cup buttermilk

3 tablespoons plain nonfat Greek yogurt

3 teaspoons fresh lemon juice

½ teaspoon kosher salt

½ teaspoon freshly ground black pepper

½ teaspoon dried oregano

½ teaspoon garlic powder

½ teaspoon onion powder

½ teaspoon dried dill

½ teaspoon sweet paprika

Pinch of cayenne (optional)

In a small bowl, combine the buttermilk, yogurt, lemon juice, salt, pepper, oregano, garlic powder, onion powder, dill, paprika, and cayenne if using. Whisk until smooth. If the dressing seems too thick, add water, 1 teaspoon at a time, until you get a consistency you like.

Tangy Five-Bean Salad Dressing

2 tablespoons olive oil

3 tablespoons apple cider vinegar

2 tablespoons sugar

4 teaspoons Dijon mustard

1 teaspoon kosher salt, plus more for seasoning

¼ teaspoon freshly ground black pepper, plus more for seasoning

Pinch of cayenne (optional)

In a small jar with a tight-fitting lid, combine the olive oil, vinegar, sugar, mustard, 1 teaspoon salt, ¼ teaspoon black pepper, and cayenne if using. Seal the jar and shake until creamy and unified, 10 to 15 seconds.

Cucumber & Hearts of Palm Salad Dressing

2 tablespoons olive oil

3 tablespoons fresh lemon juice

1 tablespoon honey

1 tablespoon Dijon mustard

¼ teaspoon kosher salt, plus more for seasoning

¼ teaspoon freshly ground black pepper, plus more for seasoning

In a medium bowl, whisk the olive oil, lemon juice, honey, mustard, salt, and pepper until creamy.

Little Gem Treasure Salad Dressing

2 tablespoons white wine vinegar

2 tablespoons olive oil

2 teaspoons finely minced shallot

1 teaspoon Dijon mustard

½ teaspoon kosher salt

½ teaspoon freshly ground black pepper

Add the vinegar, olive oil, shallot, mustard, salt, and pepper to the bowl with the orange juice. Whisk until creamy.

Mediterranean Salad Dressing

3 tablespoons red wine vinegar

2 tablespoons olive oil

1 tablespoon chopped fresh jalapeño (seeds removed to reduce heat, if desired)

1 garlic clove, minced

1 teaspoon dried oregano

½ teaspoon kosher salt

½ teaspoon ground coriander

In a large bowl, whisk together the vinegar, olive oil, jalapeño, garlic, oregano, salt, and coriander.

Creamy Lemon Dressing

⅔ cup chopped silken tofu

⅓ cup fresh lemon juice

2 tablespoons olive oil

1 teaspoon grainy or brown Dijon mustard

½ teaspoon salt

¼ teaspoon freshly ground black pepper

2 tablespoons thinly sliced scallion greens

To a blender, add the tofu, lemon juice, olive oil, mustard, salt, pepper, and scallion greens. Blend until smooth and creamy, about 20 seconds.

Creamy Mustard-Balsamic Dressing

2 tablespoons balsamic vinegar

1 tablespoon Dijon mustard

1 tablespoon olive oil

1 tablespoon water

1 garlic clove, minced

1 teaspoon kosher salt

1 teaspoon pure maple syrup

½ teaspoon freshly ground black pepper

Combine the vinegar, mustard, olive oil, water, garlic, salt, maple syrup, and black pepper in a small jar, cover tightly, and shake until creamy, about 10 seconds.

Meat and Poultry

These meaty main courses are satisfying, filling, and yet they are less calorie dense and more nutrient rich than your typical meat-and-potatoes fare. You can still eat meat and feel satisfied with these lightened-up recipes.

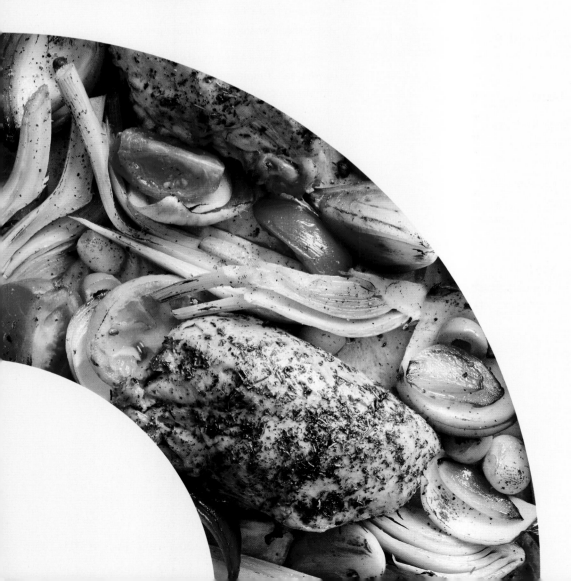

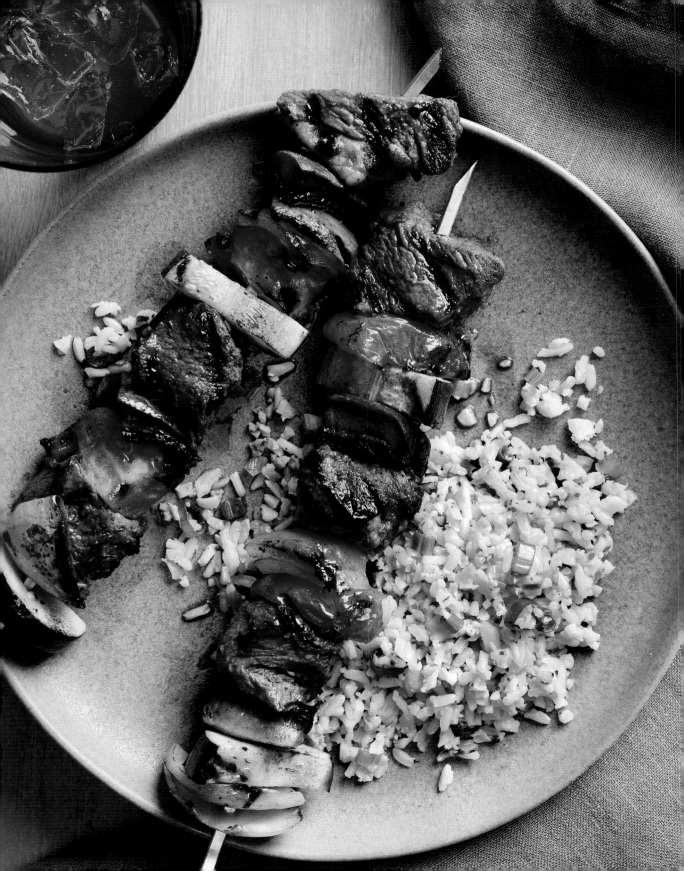

Beefy Shish Kabobs

Isn't food more fun when it's served on a stick? These beef kabobs (sometimes called kebabs) are a great way to reduce the meat portion of a meal and add more veggies. We like to serve these over Scallion-y Cauliflower & Brown Rice (page 204), but they go nicely with a salad, too.

FOR MARINATING THE MEAT

1 tablespoon olive oil

Finely grated zest and juice of 1 small lemon (about 1 teaspoon zest and 2 tablespoons juice)

2 tablespoons chopped fresh oregano

2 garlic cloves, smashed

1½ teaspoons Dijon mustard

½ teaspoon ground cumin

½ teaspoon sweet paprika

½ teaspoon kosher salt

½ teaspoon freshly ground black pepper

1 pound lean boneless sirloin (about 1 inch thick), cut into 24 1-inch cubes

FOR THE VEGGIES AND SERVING

2 medium zucchini, cut into 16 chunks

3 medium Roma (plum) tomatoes, cut into 16 chunks

1 small red onion, halved, and cut into 16 chunks

2 portobello mushroom caps, cut into 16 1-inch chunks

Kosher salt and freshly ground black pepper

Scallion-y Cauliflower & Brown Rice (optional; page 204)

SERVES 4 TOTAL TIME: 1 HOUR 20 MINUTES (INCLUDING MARINATING)

1. Prepare the meat and skewers: In a medium bowl, combine the olive oil with the lemon zest and juice, oregano, garlic, mustard, cumin, paprika, and salt and pepper. Add the meat cubes, toss to coat well, cover, and marinate on the counter for 1 hour (or in the refrigerator for up to 24 hours).

2. Soak 8 10-inch wooden skewers in water for at least 30 minutes (or use metal skewers).

3. Assemble and grill the kabobs: Heat a grill to medium hot or preheat a stovetop grill pan over medium-high heat.

4. Working in whatever order you want, thread 3 cubes of meat and 2 cubes each of the zucchini, tomatoes, red onion, and mushrooms on each skewer. Season generously with salt and pepper.

5. Place the kabobs on the grill and cook, turning every 2 minutes, until the meat and vegetables are lightly charred, the vegetables are tender, and the meat is cooked to medium-rare, about 8 minutes total.

6. Serve the kabobs: Put 2 skewers on each of 4 plates and serve, if desired, with the cauliflower and rice side dish.

NUTRITIONAL INFORMATION (1 SERVING = 2 KABOBS) Calories 230, Total Fat 8.6 g 13%, Saturated Fat 2.3 g 12%, Trans Fat 0.0 g, Cholesterol 68 mg 23%, Sodium 303.4 mg 13%, Total Carb 11.2 g 4%, Dietary Fiber 3.4 g 13%, Sugars 5.5 g, Added Sugars 0 g, Protein 28.1 g 56%, Vitamin D 6.5 mcg 2%, Calcium 78.8 mg 8%, Iron 3.1 mg 17%, Potassium 959.5 mg 27%

Chicken Tagine

A tagine is both a Moroccan stew and the unusual pot with the cone-shaped lid that is classically used to prepare the stew. Any pot will serve for cooking this delicious stew; what matters are the ingredients—tender chicken, highly flavored spices, tasty veggies chickpeas, and the sweetness of dried fruits, all of which make this a truly special meal.

FOR THE CHICKEN

6 small boneless, skinless chicken thighs (1½ pounds total)

½ teaspoon kosher salt

1 tablespoon olive oil

FOR THE SAUCE

1 medium onion, thinly sliced

4 large garlic cloves, minced

1 tablespoon minced fresh ginger

1 teaspoon ground cinnamon

1 teaspoon ground turmeric

1 teaspoon ground cumin

¼ teaspoon freshly ground black pepper

½ teaspoon ground cardamom

¼ cup red pepper flakes

½ teaspoon kosher salt

FOR THE TAGINE

3 cups reduced-sodium chicken broth

1 15-ounce can chickpeas, drained and rinsed

1 medium zucchini, halved lengthwise and cut into 1½-inch pieces

1 medium carrot, cut on the diagonal into 1-inch pieces

6 dried apricots, halved

6 pitted prunes, halved

FOR SERVING

Kosher salt

¼ cup chopped fresh cilantro

SERVES 6   TOTAL TIME: 1 HOUR

1. Cook the chicken: Season the chicken on both sides with the salt.

2. Heat the olive oil in a large (at least 6-quart) heavy-bottomed pot over medium-high heat.

3. Add the chicken and cook until golden on one side, 4 to 5 minutes. Flip over and cook until golden on the other side, another 3 minutes.

4. Transfer the chicken to a plate and cover to keep warm. (It doesn't have to be cooked through yet.)

5. Make the sauce: Reduce the heat under the pot to low and add the onion. Cook, stirring, until lightly golden, 7 to 8 minutes. Add the garlic and ginger and cook, stirring often, until fragrant, 2 minutes. Stir in the cinnamon, turmeric, cumin, black pepper, cardamom, red pepper flakes, and salt.

6. Assemble the tagine: Return the chicken to the pot and add the broth, chickpeas, zucchini, carrot, apricots, and prunes. Raise the heat to medium-high, bring to a boil, reduce the heat to medium-low, cover, and cook until the chicken is tender, about 30 minutes. Remove the lid and continue to cook until the liquid has slightly thickened, about 5 minutes more.

7. Serve the tagine: Remove the pot from the heat, season to taste with salt, and divide the tagine among 6 bowls. Garnish each bowl with some of the cilantro and serve hot.

NUTRITIONAL INFORMATION (1 SERVING = 1 CHICKEN THIGH, PLUS 1 CUP VEGETABLES)
Calories 294, Total Fat 7.7 g 12%, Saturated Fat 1.6 g 8%, Trans Fat 0.2 g, Cholesterol 94.1 mg 31%, Sodium 837.7 mg 35%, Total Carb 29.3 g 10%, Dietary Fiber 5.3 g 21%, Sugars 8.1 g, Added Sugars 0 g, Protein 27.4 g 55%, Vitamin D 5.7 mcg 1%, Calcium 62.5 mg 6%, Iron 2.8 mg 15%, Potassium 663.4 mg 19%

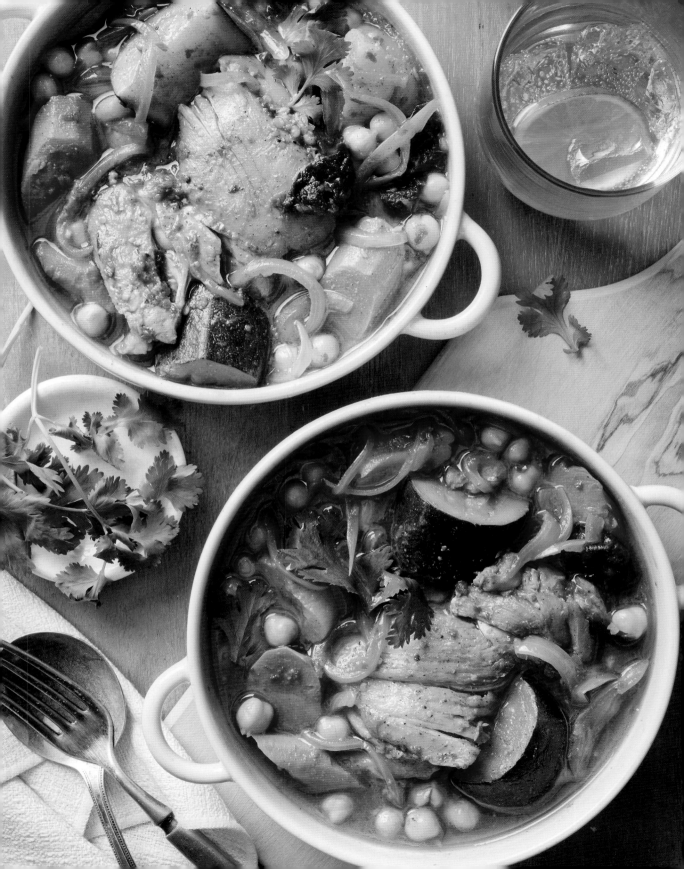

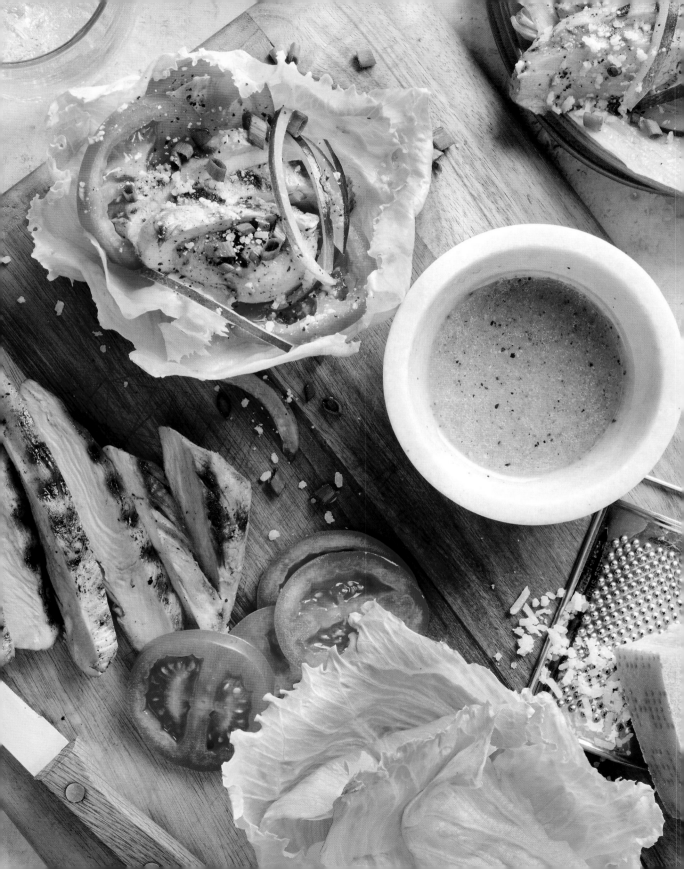

Chicken Caesar Lettuce Wraps

A wrap doesn't have to involve a big, flavorless, floury tortilla. Crunchy iceberg lettuce makes a superior wrap that is much less calorically dense and won't disintegrate as it soaks up this yummy dressing.

FOR THE DRESSING

2 tablespoons olive oil

2 tablespoons fresh lemon juice

1 tablespoon finely grated Parmigiano-Reggiano cheese

½ teaspoon Dijon mustard

½ teaspoon Worcestershire sauce

½ teaspoon fish sauce

½ teaspoon kosher salt

½ teaspoon freshly ground black pepper

FOR THE CHICKEN AND WRAPS

1 head iceberg lettuce

Olive oil cooking spray

4 4-ounce very thin chicken cutlets

2 ripe medium tomatoes, each sliced into 6 rounds

¼ cup sliced red onion

¼ cup thin Parmigiano-Reggiano cheese shavings

¼ cup thinly sliced scallion greens

Salt and freshly ground black pepper

SERVES 4 TOTAL TIME: 25 MINUTES

1. Make the dressing: In a small bowl, whisk together the olive oil, lemon juice, grated cheese, mustard, Worcestershire sauce, fish sauce, salt, and pepper until fully incorporated.

2. Prepare the lettuce wraps: Use a small knife to cut the core from the lettuce. Gently separate the leaves until you have 8 large leaves suitable for wrapping.

3. Place 4 smaller leaves inside the larger ones to form double-layered wraps.

4. Grill the chicken: Heat a grill to very hot or preheat a stovetop grill pan over high heat.

5. Measure 2 tablespoons of the dressing into a small bowl and brush it all over the chicken.

6. Grill the chicken until grill marks form and the chicken is cooked through, 2 to 3 minutes per side (or a bit more if the chicken is thicker; check for doneness). Let the chicken rest for 5 minutes.

7. Assemble the wraps: Lay 1 cutlet on each of the lettuce wraps. Layer each wrap with 3 tomato slices, 1 tablespoon of red onion, and 1 tablespoon of cheese shavings. Drizzle each wrap with 1½ teaspoons of the dressing and 1 tablespoon of the scallion greens. Season to taste with salt and pepper, and serve warm or at room temperature.

Note: You could also wrap these in plastic or foil and enjoy them chilled. They'll last for about 1 day in the refrigerator.

NUTRITIONAL INFORMATION (1 SERVING = 1 WRAP) Calories 303, Total Fat 12.8 g 20%, Saturated Fat 3.6 g 18%, Trans Fat 0.0 g, Cholesterol 136.2 mg 45%, Sodium 507.6 mg 21%, Total Carb 8.8 g 3%, Dietary Fiber 2.8 g 11%, Sugars 5.2 g, Added Sugars 0 g, Protein 40.3 g 81%, Vitamin D 1.1 mcg 0%, Calcium 119.8 mg 12%, Iron 1.5 mg 8%, Potassium 756.9 mg 22%

Grilled Sirloin Salad

This tasty salad is full of smoky flavors—you grill the steak, tomatoes, and onions all together before piling them into a salad to enjoy. Tastes like summer, all year round.

FOR THE GRILLING

1 pound lean boneless sirloin steak, patted dry

4 ripe medium Roma (plum) tomatoes, cored and halved

4 scallions, trimmed

1 tablespoon olive oil

Kosher salt and freshly ground black pepper

FOR THE VINAIGRETTE

3 tablespoons olive oil

1½ tablespoons sherry vinegar

¼ teaspoon ground cumin

Pinch of cayenne

¼ teaspoon kosher salt

¼ teaspoon freshly ground black pepper

FOR THE SALAD

2 romaine hearts (about 10 ounces total), chopped (about 8 cups)

Kosher salt and freshly ground black pepper

SERVES 4   TOTAL TIME: 30 MINUTES

1. Grill the steak, tomatoes, and scallions: Let the steak come to room temperature on the counter for 15 to 20 minutes.

2. Heat a grill to medium-hot or preheat a stovetop grill pan over medium-high heat.

3. On a cutting board, brush the tomatoes and scallions with the olive oil.

4. Season the steak, scallions, and cut sides of the tomatoes with a little salt and pepper.

5. Arrange the steak on the grill and add the tomatoes, cut sides down. Arrange the scallions crosswise over the grill grates.

6. After grilling for about 6 minutes, transfer the tomatoes and scallions to a tray; they should be lightly charred and softened.

7. Flip the steak and continue to grill until an instant-read thermometer inserted into the thickest part reaches 125°F for medium rare. This should take another 4 minutes or so. Transfer the steak to a cutting board to rest.

8. Make the vinaigrette: While the steak is resting, chop the scallion greens into 1-inch lengths and finely chop the scallion whites. Add them both to a small bowl and add the olive oil, vinegar, cumin, cayenne, salt, and pepper.

9. Assemble the dish: Arrange the romaine on a large serving platter. Thinly slice the steak across the grain, then arrange on top of the lettuce. Quarter the tomatoes and arrange them on the lettuce as well. Drizzle the vinaigrette over the salad and season generously to taste with salt and pepper. Serve family style.

NUTRITIONAL INFORMATION (1 SERVING = ¼ STEAK, PLUS 3 CUPS SALAD) Calories 300, Total Fat 18.6 g 29%, Saturated Fat 3.6 g 18%, Trans Fat 0.0 g, Cholesterol 68 mg 23%, Sodium 169.4 mg 7%, Total Carb 6.7 g 2%, Dietary Fiber 3.2 g 13%, Sugars 3.1 g, Added Sugars 0 g, Protein 27.1 g 54%, Vitamin D 2.3 mcg 1%, Calcium 77.2 mg 8%, Iron 3.2 mg 18%, Potassium 819 mg 23%

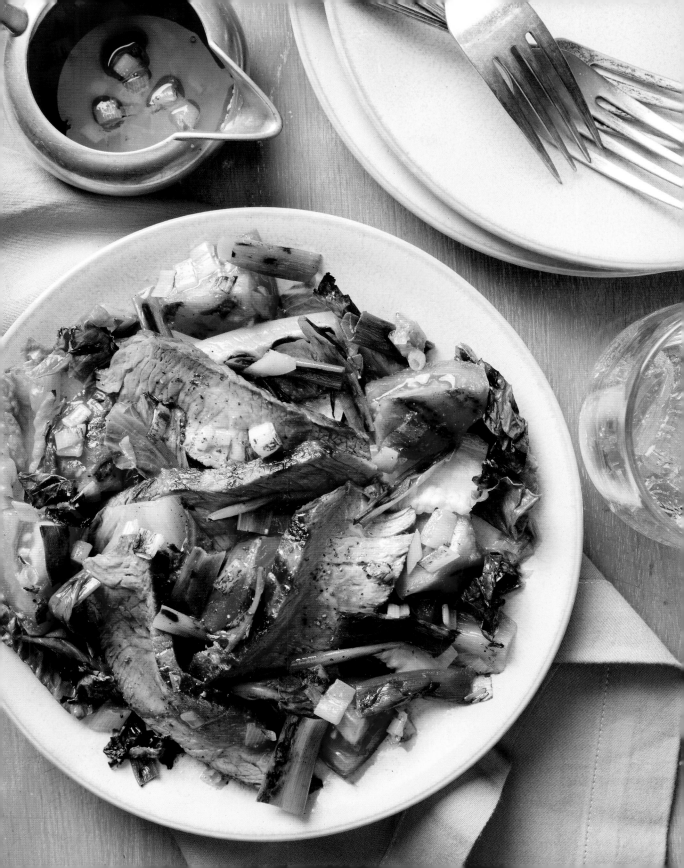

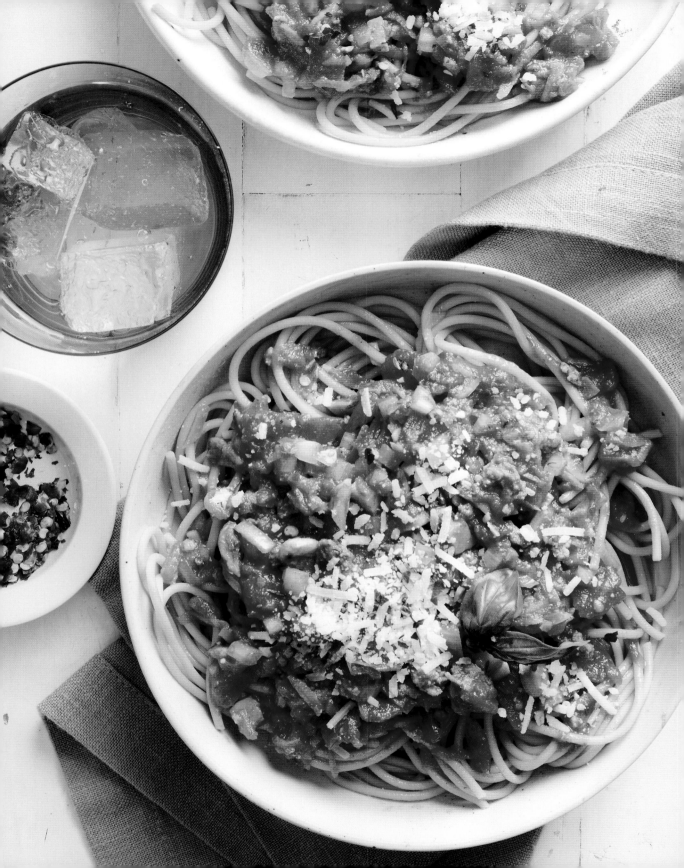

Hearty Turkey Bolognese

A meaty Bolognese sauce just might be the most popular topping for spaghetti, but it's calorically dense. This lighter version uses ground turkey and fiber-rich spelt spaghetti for more nutrients, but it's got all the pleasure, flavor, and texture of the traditional dish.

FOR THE TURKEY

Olive oil cooking spray

1¼ pounds ground turkey (93 percent lean)

¾ teaspoons kosher salt

¼ teaspoon freshly ground black pepper

FOR THE SAUCE

1 tablespoon olive oil

1 large onion, finely diced

3 garlic cloves, minced

1 8-ounce package white button mushrooms, stem ends trimmed, caps very finely chopped

2 tablespoons tomato paste

2 small carrots, grated

1 large celery stalk, diced

1 bay leaf

1 teaspoon dried thyme

1 teaspoon sweet paprika

¾ teaspoon kosher salt, plus more for seasoning

½ teaspoon freshly ground black pepper, plus more for seasoning

¼ teaspoon red pepper flakes (optional)

1 28-ounce can crushed tomatoes

1 14-ounce can petite diced tomatoes

2 cups water

1 teaspoon red wine vinegar

FOR THE PASTA AND TO SERVE

Kosher salt

1 pound spelt spaghetti (or other whole-grain spaghetti)

½ cup finely grated Parmigiano-Reggiano cheese

Chopped fresh basil, for garnish

SERVES 8 TOTAL TIME: 1 HOUR 15 MINUTES

1. Cook the turkey: Spray a large (at least 5-quart) saucepan or Dutch oven with the olive oil cooking spray and place over medium heat. Add the turkey, salt, and pepper. Cook, stirring often and breaking up the meat with a spoon, until the turkey is opaque and just cooked through, 5 to 6 minutes. Transfer to a medium bowl.

2. Make the sauce: Add the olive oil to the pot, then add the onion and cook, stirring frequently, until lightly golden, 6 to 7 minutes. Add the garlic and cook, stirring, for 1 more minute.

3. Add the mushrooms and cook, stirring frequently, until they release their water, 5 to 6 minutes. Add the tomato paste and cook, stirring, 1 more minute.

4. Add the carrots, celery, bay leaf, thyme, paprika, ¾ teaspoon salt, ½ teaspoon pepper, and red pepper flakes, if using. Cook, stirring, until the vegetables begin to soften, about 5 minutes.

5. Add the crushed and diced tomatoes with their juices, the water, and the vinegar. Bring to a boil, reduce the heat to medium-low, and simmer, stirring occasionally, until the sauce thickens and darkens slightly in color, 30 to 35 minutes.

6. Season to taste with additional salt and pepper.

continued on page 124

continued from page 123

7. Make the pasta: While the sauce is simmering, bring a large (at least 6-quart) pot of generously salted water (about 1 teaspoon per quart of water) to a boil. Add the pasta and cook until al dente, following the package directions.

8. Assemble and serve the spaghetti: Portion 1 cup of cooked pasta into each of 8 bowls, then top each with 1 cup sauce, 1 tablespoon cheese, and a sprinkling of basil. Serve hot.

NUTRITIONAL INFORMATION (1 SERVING = 1 CUP SPAGHETTI, 1 CUP SAUCE, AND 1 TABLESPOON CHEESE) Calories 405, Total Fat 11.6 g 18%, Saturated Fat 3.4 g 17%, Trans Fat 0.5 g, Cholesterol 58.1 mg 19%, Sodium 627.3 mg 26%, Total Carb 54.2 g 18%, Dietary Fiber 8.7 g 35%, Sugars 12.2 g, Added Sugars 0 g, Protein 27 g 54%, Vitamin D 11.9 mcg 3%, Calcium 154.9 mg 15%, Iron 4.7 mg 26%, Potassium 895.3 mg 26%

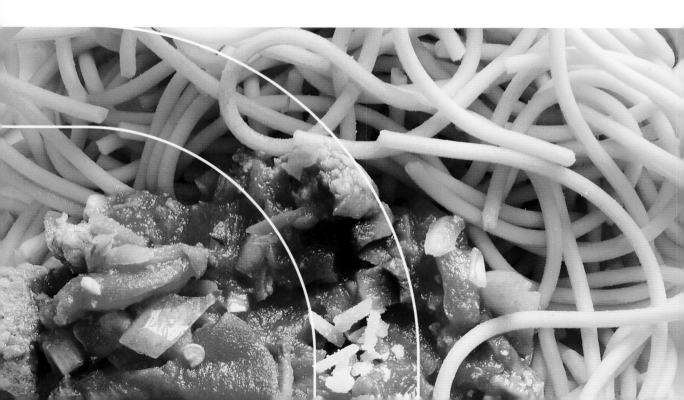

Sheet-Pan Chicken & Vegetables

Sheet-pan (rimmed baking sheet) recipes are great for varying recipe flavor profiles. This recipe has a Mediterranean profile, with its fennel, tomatoes, garlic, olives, capers, and herbs. But you could easily change this by substituting veggies, herbs, and spices from other cuisines. For instance, you could give this dish an Asian profile by substituting bok choy, scallions, snow peas, napa cabbage, and shiitake mushrooms, along with some five-spice powder or fresh Thai basil. Or you could give this dish a Latin profile by using yellow squash, zucchini, corn, jalapeños, fresh cilantro, and chipotle chile powder. We love meals that are this flexible!

FOR THE VEGETABLES AND CHICKEN

2 medium fennel bulbs (about 1 pound)

4 medium tomatoes, cut into 8 wedges

1 medium red onion, cut into 8 wedges

1 lemon, thinly sliced, seeds removed

10 pitted green olives, such as Castelvetrano, halved

10 small garlic cloves

2 tablespoons drained and rinsed capers

1 tablespoon olive oil

½ teaspoon kosher salt

¼ teaspoon freshly ground black pepper

2 large bone-in chicken breasts (about 2 pounds total), skin removed

FOR THE HERB PASTE

1 tablespoon olive oil

½ teaspoon dried basil

½ teaspoon dried thyme

½ teaspoon dried oregano

½ teaspoon kosher salt

¼ teaspoon freshly ground black pepper

FOR SERVING

Kosher salt and freshly ground black pepper

1 lemon, cut into 4 wedges

SERVES 4   TOTAL TIME: 1 HOUR 5 MINUTES

1. Preheat the oven to 425°F.

2. Prepare the vegetables: Cut off the feathery fronds from the fennel bulbs and discard. Peel off the tough outer layers of the bulbs, then cut the bulbs in half lengthwise. Use a paring knife to cut out and discard the V-shaped small white core, then cut each fennel half into 4 wedges.

3. Place the fennel wedges in a large bowl and add the tomatoes, onion, lemon slices, olives, garlic, capers, olive oil, salt, and black pepper. Toss gently to coat the vegetables with the seasonings.

4. Prepare the sheet pan: Line a rimmed baking sheet with parchment. Spread the vegetables on the baking sheet, then nestle the chicken breasts in the center of the vegetables.

5. Make the herb paste: In a small bowl, combine the oil with the basil, thyme, oregano, salt, and pepper. Rub the tops of the chicken breasts with the herb paste.

6. Bake the dish: Place a piece of parchment on the chicken, then cover the baking sheet with foil. Bake until the fennel and onion pieces begin to soften, 25 to 30 minutes.

continued on page 127

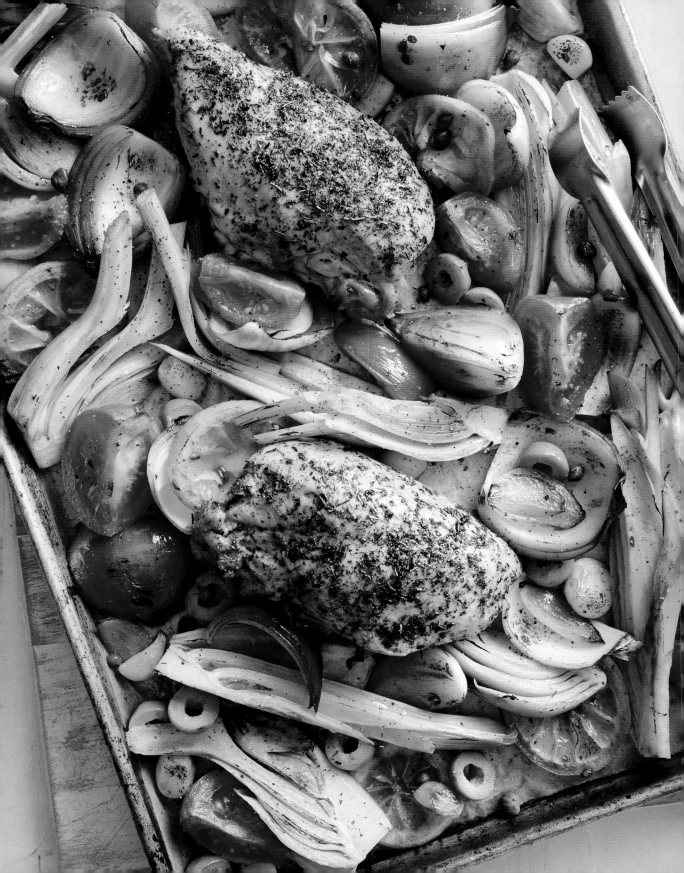

continued from page 125

7. Briefly take the baking sheet out of the oven. Uncover the chicken breasts. Reduce the oven to 400°F and place the baking sheet back in the oven. Continue to bake until the fennel pieces are tender and the onion and lemon slices are lightly caramelized, 25 to 30 minutes.

8. Serve the dish: Let the chicken rest for 5 minutes, then cut each breast in half with a cleaver (or slice the meat from the bone and then cut in half). Place the chicken pieces on a large platter, spread the vegetables around them, and drizzle any pan juices on top. Season to taste with salt and pepper. Serve family style, with lemon wedges.

NUTRITIONAL INFORMATION (1 SERVING = ½ CHICKEN BREAST AND 1¼ CUPS VEGETABLES) Calories 405, Total Fat 21.9 g 34%, Saturated Fat 5.1 g 26%, Trans Fat 0.2 g, Cholesterol 92.8 mg 31%, Sodium 762.7 mg 32%, Total Carb 20.7 g 7%, Dietary Fiber 6.7 g 27%, Sugars 9.1 g, Added Sugars 0 g, Protein 34 g 68%, Vitamin D 23.2 mcg 6%, Calcium 117.2 mg 12%, Iron 3 mg 16%, Potassium 1102.2 mg 31%

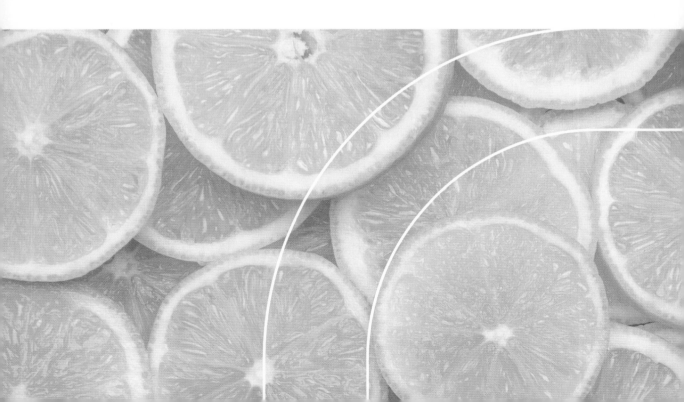

Orange Beef Stir-Fry

The sweet orange sauce brings out the flavors of the meat and vegetables, and this version is lighter, less greasy, and fresher than what you could order in. If you want to skip the rice, serve this with extra broccoli or those nifty shirataki noodles.

FOR SEASONING THE STEAK

12 ounces lean boneless sirloin steak

1 tablespoon low-sodium soy sauce

1 teaspoon toasted sesame oil

FOR THE SAUCE

1 large orange

¾ cup low-sodium chicken broth

2 tablespoons cornstarch

1 tablespoon low-sodium soy sauce

1 teaspoon toasted sesame oil

1 teaspoon unseasoned rice vinegar

FOR THE STIR-FRY AND SERVING

1 tablespoon vegetable oil

1 small red onion, cut into 1-inch chunks

4 cups broccoli florets

1 red bell pepper, cored, seeded, and cut into 1-inch pieces

1 8-ounce package white button mushrooms, trimmed and quartered

4 scallions, thinly sliced, white and green parts kept separate

2 cups cooked jasmine brown rice, warmed

SERVES 6 TOTAL TIME: 1 HOUR (INCLUDING FREEZING)

1. Prepare the steak: Wrap the sirloin well in plastic wrap and freeze for 30 minutes.

2. Remove the steak from the freezer, unwrap, and use a sharp knife to slice it across the grain into very thin slices. Place the slices in a medium bowl. Add the soy sauce and sesame oil and toss to coat.

3. Prepare the sauce: Remove thick strips of zest from the orange. Juice the orange; you should have about ½ cup juice. Place the zest strips and juice in a medium bowl. Add the broth, cornstarch, soy sauce, sesame oil, and vinegar. Whisk to combine.

4. Cook the steak: Heat a large (12-inch) skillet or wok over medium-high heat. When very hot, add 1½ teaspoons of the oil and use a heatproof pastry brush to spread the oil around. Use tongs to add half the meat slices in a single layer to the skillet. Cook until the meat is seared and just barely cooked through, about 2 minutes per side.

5. Transfer the meat to a plate. Repeat with the remaining slices.

6. Cook the vegetables: Add the remaining 1½ teaspoons oil to the skillet, then add the red onion. Stir-fry, scraping up the browned bits from the pan, until the onion softens but retains some crunch, 2 to 3 minutes.

7. Add the broccoli, red pepper, mushrooms, and scallion whites. Cover and steam until the broccoli turns bright green, 2 to 3 minutes.

8. Combine the stir-fry: Whisk the sauce, then drizzle it into the skillet and quickly add the orange zest and the steak slices. Stir to incorporate, then cook until the sauce is bubbling and has thickened, 2 to 3 minutes. Stir in most of the scallion greens.

9. Serve the stir-fry: Spoon ⅓ cup rice into each of 6 bowls. Spoon about 1½ cups of the stir-fry along with some of the sauce into each bowl, and garnish with the remaining scallion greens.

NUTRITIONAL INFORMATION (1 SERVING = 1½ CUPS STIR-FRY, WITH ⅓ CUP RICE)
Calories 304, Total Fat 13.1 g 20%, Saturated Fat 3.8 g 19%, Trans Fat 0.0 g, Cholesterol 44.2 mg 15%, Sodium 240.7 mg 10%, Total Carb 30.5 g 10%, Dietary Fiber 4.2 g 17%, Sugars 6.3 g, Added Sugars 0 g, Protein 17.9 g 36%, Vitamin D 2.7 mcg 1%, Calcium 69.6 mg 7%, Iron 2.2 mg 12%, Potassium 687.7 mg 20%

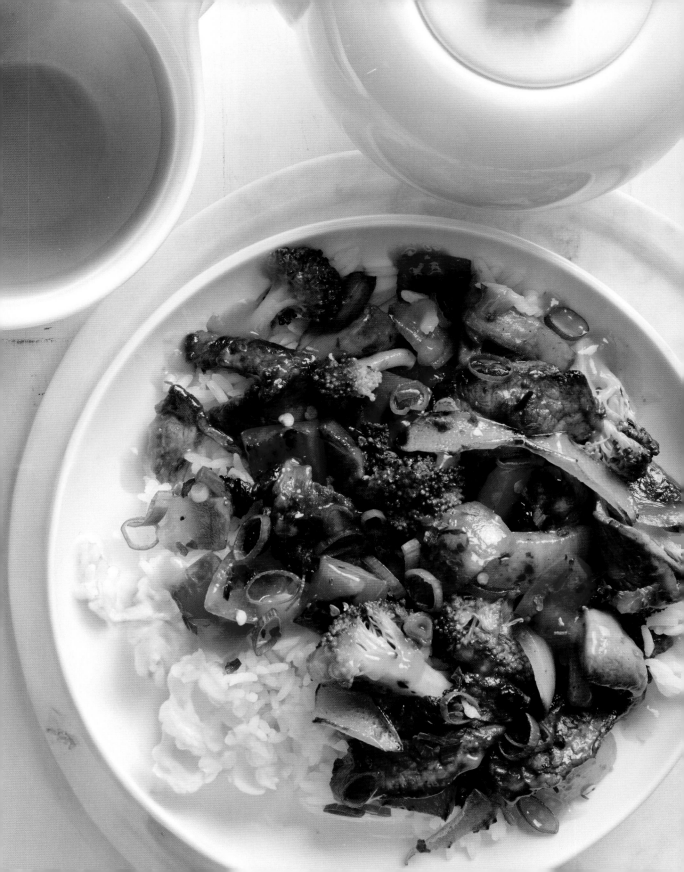

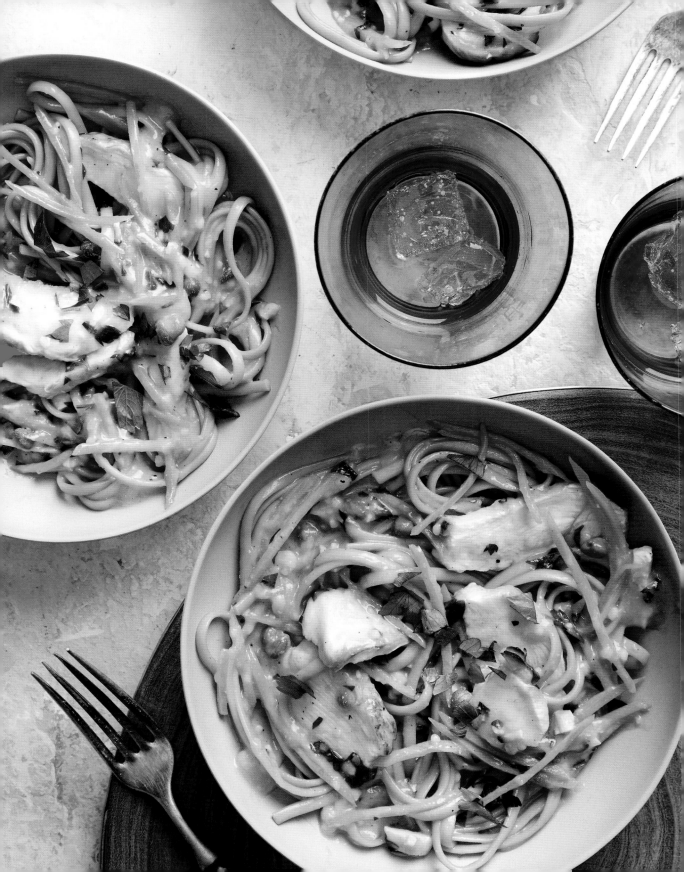

Chicken Piccata Pasta

Buttery, briny chicken piccata is a classic Italian dish. We've lightened it up by significantly reducing the fat without sacrificing any of the flavor. Note: As an alternative to using the peeler, you could grate the carrots on a box grater; you'll need 2½ cups grated carrots.

SERVES 4 TOTAL TIME: 50 MINUTES

FOR THE PASTA AND CHICKEN

Kosher salt

6 ounces whole wheat linguine

1 pound thin chicken cutlets

½ tablespoon finely grated lemon zest

½ tablespoon fresh lemon juice

1 tablespoon olive oil

½ teaspoon freshly ground black pepper

FOR THE SAUCE

2 cups low-sodium chicken broth, chilled

2 tablespoons cornstarch

1 tablespoon olive oil

3 garlic cloves, minced

2 large, preferably long carrots, cut into long, thin strips with a Y-peeler (see Note)

FOR ASSEMBLING AND SERVING

2 tablespoons drained and rinsed capers

¼ cup chopped fresh parsley, plus more for garnish

½ tablespoon finely grated lemon zest

3½ tablespoons fresh lemon juice

½ cup finely grated Parmigiano-Reggiano cheese

½ teaspoon kosher salt

¼ teaspoon freshly ground black pepper

1. Cook the pasta: Fill a large (at least 6-quart) pot with water and add salt (about 1 teaspoon salt per quart). Bring to a boil, add the pasta, and cook until al dente, according to package directions. Drain the pasta in a colander, reserving 1 cup of the pasta water.

2. Prepare the chicken: While the pasta is cooking, in a large bowl, combine the chicken, lemon zest and lemon juice, ½ teaspoon salt, and the black pepper and toss to coat well.

3. Heat the olive oil in a large (12-inch) skillet over medium-high heat. Add the chicken and cook, not moving it, until lightly golden, 2 to 3 minutes, then flip and cook the other side. Transfer the chicken to a cutting board. Let rest 5 minutes, then slice crosswise into ½-inch strips. Cover with foil to keep warm.

4. Cook the sauce: In a small bowl, whisk together the broth and cornstarch until dissolved.

5. Place the skillet over medium-low heat and add the oil. Add the garlic and cook, stirring, until fragrant, 1 minute. Add the carrot strips and the cornstarch mixture, raise the heat to medium-high, bring to a boil, and cook, stirring and scraping up any browned bits with a wooden spoon, just until the liquid thickens and the carrots soften, 2 to 3 minutes.

6. Assemble the dish and serve: Return the pasta to the pot along with the chicken strips. Add the capers and toss to coat.

7. Stir in the parsley, lemon zest and lemon juice, Parmigiano-Reggiano, salt, and pepper. Cook until all ingredients are warmed through, 3 to 5 minutes, adding the reserved pasta water by the tablespoon as needed.

continued on page 132

continued from page 131

8. Divide the mixture among 4 pasta bowls and garnish each with some more parsley. Serve hot.

NUTRITIONAL INFORMATION (1 SERVING = 1½ CUPS CHICKEN, PASTA, AND VEGETABLES)
Calories 330, Total Fat 13.7 g 21%, Saturated Fat 4.3 g 22%, Trans Fat 0.0 g, Cholesterol 23.8 mg 8%, Sodium 672.2 mg 28%, Total Carb 42 g 14%, Dietary Fiber 6.1 g 25%, Sugars 2.4 g, Added Sugars 0 g, Protein 16.7 g 33%, Vitamin D 0.9 mcg 0%, Calcium 197.8 mg 20%, Iron 2.2 mg 12%, Potassium 337.7 mg 10%

NOOM CHEF'S TIP: MAKING A PERFECT CORNSTARCH SLURRY
An easy way to thicken cooking liquids like sauces without adding extra butter is to make a cornstarch slurry, which is a mixture of water (or broth) and cornstarch. If you have time, put your liquid in the refrigerator for a few hours before making the slurry—this will help the cornstarch dissolve better. Whisk the cornstarch into the cold liquid at a ratio of approximately 1 or 2 tablespoons cornstarch per 1 cup of liquid, until the cornstarch is completely dissolved. Then, whisk the slurry into the hot soup, stew, or sauce as it cooks, and keep stirring—the liquid will thicken rapidly. This trick works for just about any soup, stew, sauce, or gravy.

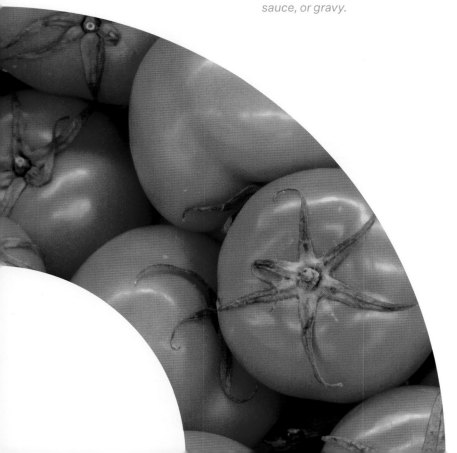

Saucy Pizza-Stuffed Chicken Breasts

Want a filling meal that gives you all the flavors of pizza with tons of protein? Yes, please! We think you'll love the saucy flavor of these chicken breasts stuffed with pizza filling. Choose thick chicken breasts for this recipe, and be careful when cutting the pocket into each breast. You may prefer to cut them when the chicken isn't quite completely thawed, so the meat is firmer and easier to cut—just watch your fingers!

FOR THE SAUCE

1 tablespoon olive oil

1 medium onion, chopped

1½ tablespoons water

1 large garlic clove, minced

1 tablespoon tomato paste

1 14-ounce can crushed tomatoes

2 teaspoons dried oregano

½ teaspoon kosher salt

½ teaspoon red wine vinegar

FOR THE FILLING

5 ounces fresh baby spinach leaves, large stems removed

½ cup shredded part-skim mozzarella cheese

¼ cup finely grated Parmigiano-Reggiano cheese

1 ounce thinly sliced pepperoni, finely chopped

1 teaspoon finely minced garlic

1 teaspoon dried oregano

1 teaspoon sweet paprika

¼ teaspoon freshly ground black pepper

¼ to ½ teaspoon red pepper flakes

FOR BAKING AND SERVING

2 large (8-ounce) boneless, skinless chicken breasts

Salt and freshly ground black pepper

2 teaspoons olive oil

2 tablespoons shredded mozzarella

Sweet paprika

Chopped fresh basil

SERVES 4 TOTAL TIME: 1 HOUR

1. Make the sauce: Heat the olive oil in a small saucepan over medium heat. Add the onion and cook, stirring, until lightly golden, 8 to 9 minutes, adding the water after 5 minutes to prevent the onion from sticking. Continue to cook for about 8 to 9 minutes total.

2. Add the garlic and continue to cook, stirring, for 1 more minute. Add the tomato paste and cook, stirring, for another minute, then add the crushed tomatoes, oregano, salt, and vinegar.

3. Bring to a low boil over medium heat, then reduce the heat to low and simmer until the sauce thickens slightly, 13 to 15 minutes, stirring frequently to prevent sticking. Remove the sauce from the heat and cover to keep warm.

4. Make the filling: Preheat the oven to 350°F.

5. Place the spinach in a large microwave-safe bowl, seal tightly, and microwave on high until the spinach is wilted, about 3 minutes. Uncover the bowl, let the spinach cool enough to handle, then squeeze out as much liquid as you can (squeeze more than you think possible).

continued on page 134

continued from page 133

6. Finely chop the spinach and put it in a bowl with the mozzarella, Parmigiano-Reggiano, pepperoni, garlic, oregano, paprika, black pepper, and red pepper flakes.

7. Stuff and bake the chicken: Using a sharp knife, cut a pocket into the side of each chicken breast that runs the length of the breast, making it as deep as you can without cutting all the way through.

8. Season the pockets with some salt and pepper, then stuff half the filling into each breast half, close it, and secure with a toothpick.

9. Arrange the chicken in a 9-inch square baking pan. Brush the chicken with the oil and sprinkle with some paprika. Bake until the chicken is just cooked through and juicy, about 25 minutes. Remove the pan and keep the oven turned on.

10. Assemble and serve the dish: Pour the sauce over the chicken breasts, then sprinkle the tops with the mozzarella. Place pan back in the oven and continue to bake until the cheese is melted and bubbly, about 5 minutes. Remove the chicken from the oven, cut into 1-inch slices, and garnish with the basil.

NUTRITIONAL INFORMATION (1 SERVING = ½ STUFFED CHICKEN BREAST) Calories 343, Total Fat 17 g 26%, Saturated Fat 5.6 g 28%, Trans Fat 0.3 g, Cholesterol 94.9 mg 32%, Sodium 896.9 mg 37%, Total Carb 14.3 g 5%, Dietary Fiber 4 g 16%, Sugars 6.2 g, Added Sugars 0 g, Protein 34.4 g 69%, Vitamin D 8.2 mcg 2%, Calcium 279.4 mg 28%, Iron 3.6 mg 20%, Potassium 1042.2 mg 30%

NOOM CHEF'S TIP: FRESH VERSUS DRIED HERBS *Fresh and dried herbs are usually interchangeable at a ratio of about 3:1, meaning that 3 parts fresh equals 1 part dried. Their flavors are similar but not exactly the same, so try both fresh and dried in your favorite recipes to see which you think goes best with what dishes. For instance, we like bright, fresh dill in soups, but we prefer more intense dried dill in our tuna salad. (We're funny that way.)*

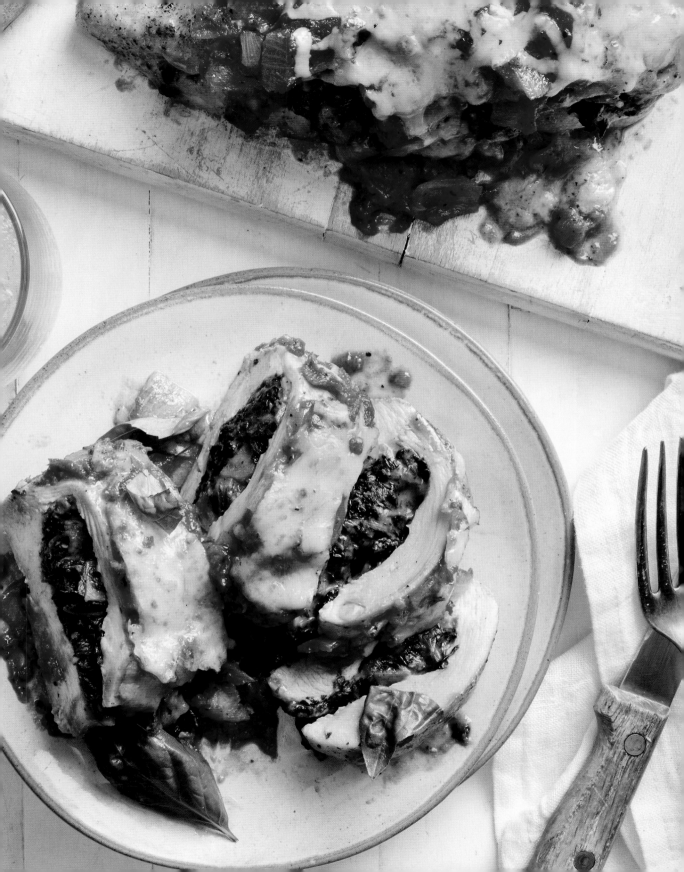

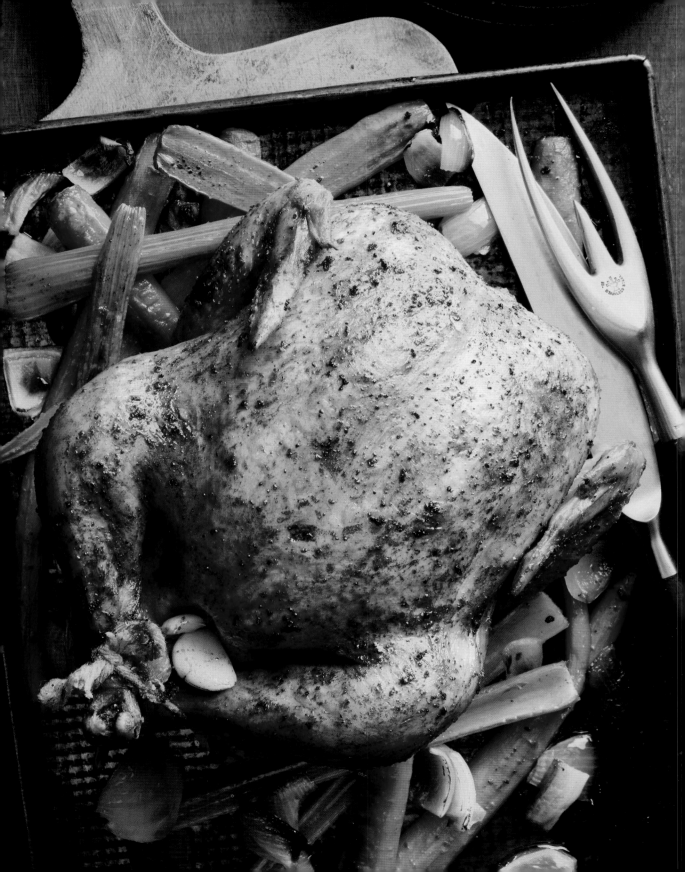

Classic Roast Chicken

Nothing says comfort food like a roasted chicken. This chicken is practically perfect for any occasion, whether you're looking to feed a crowd, have meals for the week, or prepare a cozy family dinner. You can nestle your favorite veggies to roast around the bird, and serve any of our delicious side dishes to ensure you have lots of Noomy leftovers to enjoy later in the week.

1 3½- to 4-pound roasting chicken, rinsed and patted dry

1¼ teaspoons kosher salt

½ teaspoon freshly ground black pepper

3 garlic cloves

2 tablespoons olive oil

1 teaspoon onion powder

1 teaspoon garlic powder

½ teaspoon sweet paprika

4 medium carrots, halved lengthwise

4 celery stalks, ends trimmed

1 medium onion, chopped

SERVES 6 TOTAL TIME: 1 HOUR 45 MINUTES

1. Preheat the oven to 375°F.

2. Season the chicken: Rub ¼ teaspoon each of the salt and pepper into the cavity of the chicken and place the garlic cloves inside.

3. Combine the olive oil, onion powder, garlic powder, paprika, remaining teaspoon salt, and remaining ¼ teaspoon pepper in a small bowl. Rub the spiced oil all over the chicken.

4. If you plan to carve the chicken at the table, tie the legs together with a piece of twine (this also keeps the cavity closed to better steam the garlic inside).

5. Assemble and roast: Arrange the carrots, celery, and onion in the bottom of a large roasting pan, then place the chicken on top. Roast the chicken until you can easily wiggle a leg, the juices run clear when pricked with a fork, and/or an instant-read thermometer inserted into the thickest part of the breast reads 165° F. This should take about 1½ hours.

6. Serve the chicken: Let the chicken rest for 10 minutes, then transfer it to a cutting board or carving platter and carve it, separating the wings and thighs, and slicing the 2 sides of the breast.

7. Drain the juices from the pan into a small bowl and skim off any visible fat.

8. Serve the chicken family style on a large platter, with the roasted vegetables alongside and drizzle on the chicken juices, if desired.

NUTRITIONAL INFORMATION (1 SERVING = 1 TO 2 PIECES OF CHICKEN, PLUS ⅙ OF THE VEGETABLES) Calories 404, Total Fat 27.8 g 43%, Saturated Fat 7.3 g 36%, Trans Fat 0.2 g, Cholesterol 115 mg 38%, Sodium 466.9 mg 19%, Total Carb 7.8 g 3%, Dietary Fiber 2.1 g 8%, Sugars 3.3 g, Added Sugars 0 g, Protein 29.5 g 59%, Vitamin D 15.3 mcg 4%, Calcium 51.2 mg 5%, Iron 1.8 mg 10%, Potassium 539.1 mg 15%

Open-Faced Patty Melts

For recipes that use ground meat, you may automatically reach for ground beef, but ground poultry (turkey or chicken) has less fat than standard ground beef (80 percent lean) and less saturated fat in particular. And with a recipe this tasty, you won't even notice the difference.

1 very small onion, grated or finely minced

8 ounces lean (8⅕₁₅) ground beef

8 ounces ground white-meat chicken or turkey

1 large egg white

1 teaspoon garlic powder

½ teaspoon kosher salt

½ teaspoon freshly ground black pepper

2 teaspoons vegetable oil

4 thin slices whole-grain bread (small slices, just slightly larger than a large tomato slice)

½ large ripe beefsteak tomato, cut into 4 ¼-inch-thick slices

4 very thin slices (about ½ ounce each) sharp cheddar cheese

12 bread-and-butter or dill pickle slices

SERVES 4   TOTAL TIME: 25 MINUTES

1. Prepare the meat mixture: Spread the grated onion on a small cotton kitchen towel. Roll it up, then twist to squeeze out as much liquid as you can. Add the onion to a medium bowl with the ground beef and chicken, the egg white, garlic powder, salt, and pepper. Mix well with your hands until all the ingredients are fully combined.

2. Form the meat mixture into 4 equal-sized balls (about 2 inches in diameter).

3. Cook the patties: Heat a large (12-inch), preferably cast-iron, skillet over medium-high heat. Brush the skillet with the oil, then arrange the 4 balls in the pan and press them into approximately 4-inch-round burgers.

4. Season the burgers with salt and pepper and cook, pressing down occasionally, until the underside is charred and the edges are crispy, 3 to 4 minutes. Flip the burgers and cook on the other side until lightly charred, 2 to 3 more minutes.

5. Transfer the burgers to a plate, leaving any fat in the pan.

6. Assemble and cook the sandwiches: Arrange the 4 slices of bread in the skillet. On top of each bread slice, place one of the burgers, then add a tomato slice and a slice of cheese. Cover the skillet and cook until the cheese is melted and the bottoms of the bread slices are toasted, 2 to 3 minutes. (If 4 slices of bread won't fit in your skillet and you want everything to come out hot at the same time, toast the bread and build the patty melts on a baking tray, then melt the cheese in a 350°F oven for about 10 minutes.)

7. Serve the patty melts: Remove the sandwiches to a large serving platter and top each with 3 pickle slices. Serve at once.

NUTRITIONAL INFORMATION (1 SERVING = 1 SANDWICH) Calories 388, Total Fat 17.1 g 26%, Saturated Fat 6.2 g 31%, Trans Fat 0.7 g, Cholesterol 74.8 mg 25%, Sodium 750.9 mg 31%, Total Carb 28.6 g 10%, Dietary Fiber 2.7 g 11%, Sugars 19 g, Added Sugars 0 g, Protein 25.4 g 51%, Vitamin D 8 mcg 2%, Calcium 116.8 mg 12%, Iron 2.3 mg 13%, Potassium 283.9 mg 8%

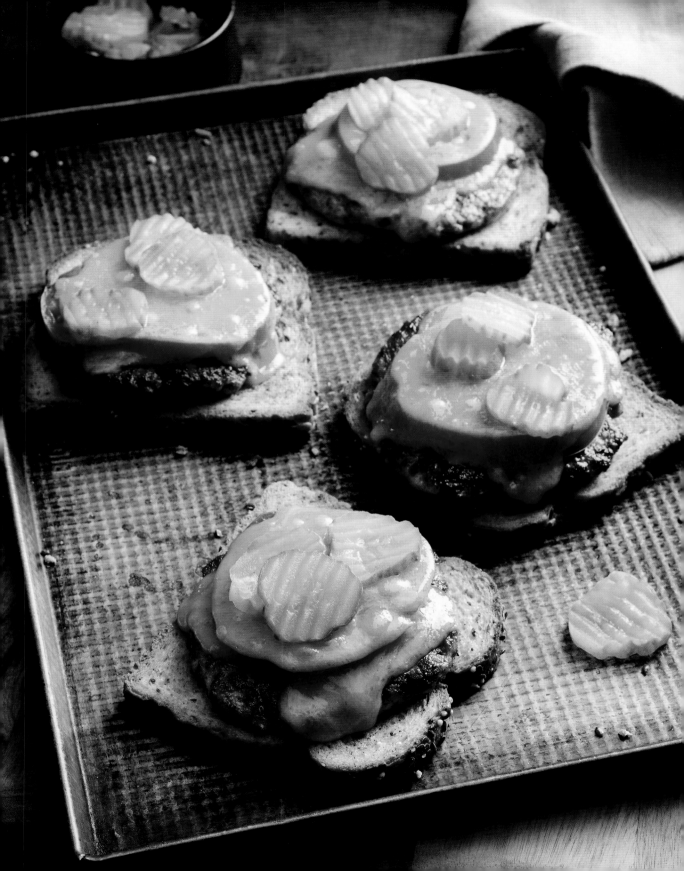

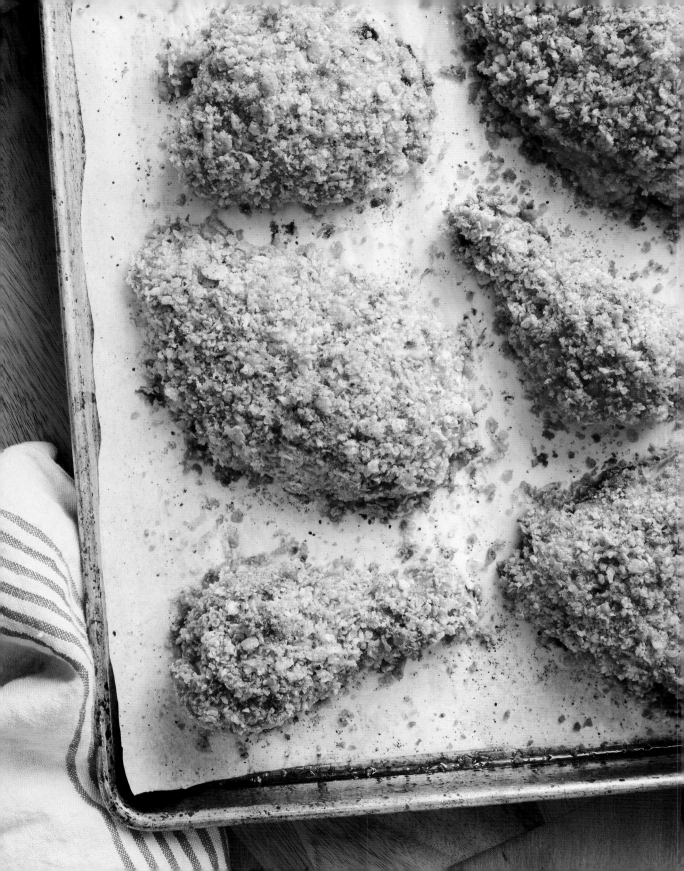

Oven "Fried" Chicken

1 small (3½- to 4-pound) whole chicken, cut into 8 pieces; or 1 package of bone-in chicken, skin removed and wings reserved for another use)

FOR THE YOGURT MIXTURE

1½ cups plain nonfat regular yogurt (not Greek)

¾ teaspoon onion powder

¾ teaspoon garlic powder

¾ teaspoon kosher salt

½ teaspoon sweet paprika

¼ teaspoon cayenne

FOR THE COATING

3 cups cornflakes cereal

1 cup panko or other bread crumbs

1 teaspoon kosher salt

1 teaspoon sweet paprika

⅛ teaspoon cayenne

FOR BAKING

Olive oil cooking spray

We love our air-fryers, but we created this oven "fried" chicken recipe to obtain the crunchy, juicy goodness of fried chicken as it comes straight out of the oven, so you can make a big batch at one time.

SERVES 4   TOTAL TIME: 1 HOUR

1. Preheat the oven to 400°F. Line a rimmed baking sheet with parchment.

2. Make the yogurt mixture: In a large bowl, whisk together the yogurt, onion powder, garlic powder, salt, paprika, and cayenne.

3. Make the coating: Process the cornflakes in a food processor until small to medium crumbs form, 15 to 20 seconds (about 2 cups crumbs). Place the crumbs in a wide, shallow bowl and stir in the panko, salt, paprika, and cayenne. Transfer half the breading (about 1 cup) to a small bowl. (If you use all the breading at once, it can get too moistened and become unusable.)

4. Bread the chicken: One at a time, dip each of the chicken pieces in the yogurt, coating each piece all over, then letting the excess drip off. Press the chicken piece into the crumbs, applying pressure to help the crumbs adhere. Gently flip and press the other side of the chicken piece into the crumbs, again applying pressure. Place the chicken piece on the baking sheet.

5. Repeat with the remaining chicken pieces, adding the reserved half of the breading to the bowl when needed. Space the chicken pieces on the baking sheet so they aren't touching.

6. Bake the chicken and serve: Spray the chicken pieces with the olive oil cooking spray, sweeping back and forth across all the pieces, for 8 seconds. Bake until the chicken is crisp and deeply golden, 35 to 40 minutes.

7. Serve the chicken hot, or cover and refrigerate the pieces and enjoy them cold the next day.

Note: The chicken will keep in the refrigerator for about 48 hours.

NUTRITIONAL INFORMATION (1 SERVING = 2 PIECES OF CHICKEN) Calories 360, Total Fat 5.5 g 8%, Saturated Fat 1.4 g 7%, Trans Fat 0.0 g, Cholesterol 123.1 mg 41%, Sodium 979.1 mg 41%, Total Carb 27.6 g 9%, Dietary Fiber 1.6 g 7%, Sugars 4.5 g, Added Sugars 0 g, Protein 48.3 g 97%, Vitamin D 30 mcg 8%, Calcium 117 mg 12%, Iron 6.3 mg 35%, Potassium 614.3 mg 18%

Seafood

The omega-3 fats in seafood are heart healthy,[1] and many experts say that eating fish and seafood twice weekly is beneficial for health.[2] Plus, seafood is delicious! Why not start eating more fish today with the tasty seafood recipes in this chapter?

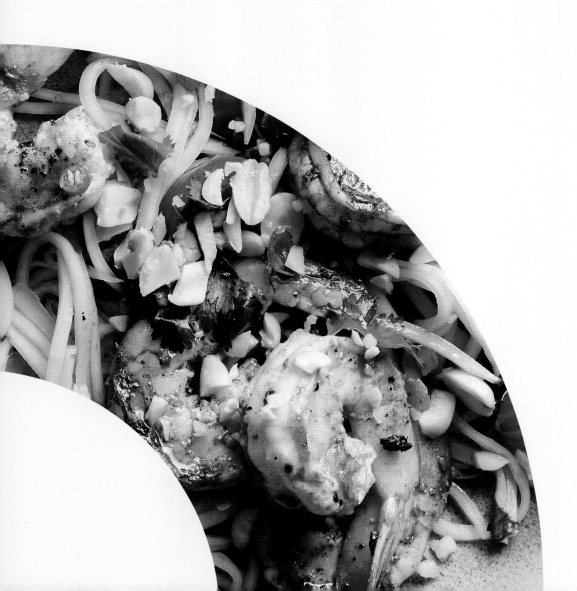

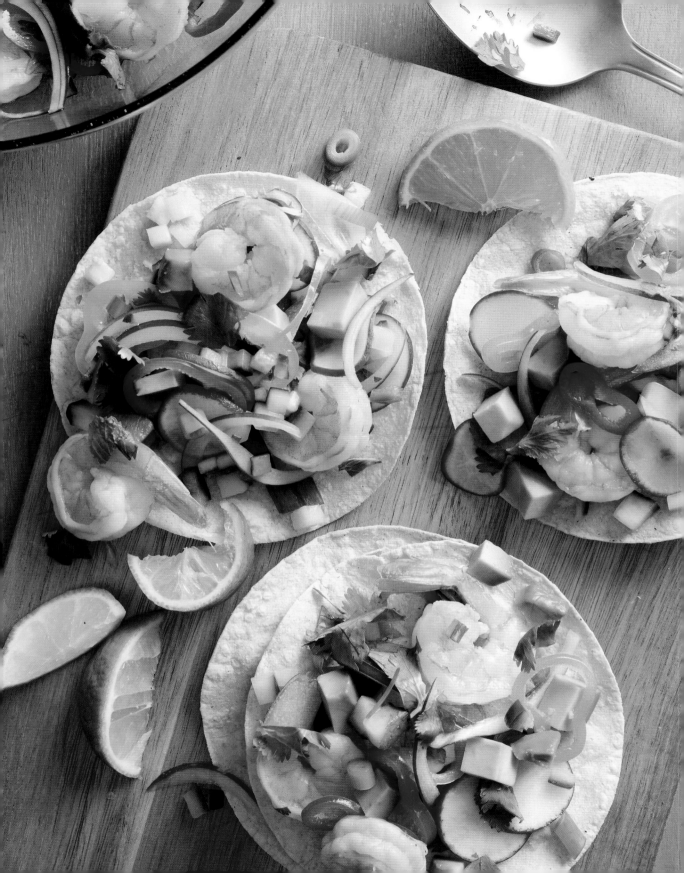

Chilled Tequila-Lime Shrimp

 This crisp, tender, refreshing dish tastes like summertime on a plate.

FOR THE MARINADE

1 cup fresh lime juice

2 tablespoons (1 ounce) tequila, or more if desired (optional)

1 tablespoon kosher salt

FOR THE CEVICHE

1 pound cooked large shrimp, shelled and cleaned

4 baby red and yellow peppers, sliced into thin rings

6 small radishes, thinly sliced

2 large Persian cucumbers, diced

½ small red onion, thinly sliced

½ cup chopped fresh cilantro

½ cup chopped scallions (green and white parts)

¼ cup chopped fresh mint

½ jalapeño, seeded if desired, sliced into thin rings

1 medium avocado, halved, pitted, and diced

FOR THE TORTILLAS

8 6-inch corn tortillas

Olive oil cooking spray

SERVES 8   TOTAL TIME: 15 MINUTES

1. Make the marinade: Combine the lime juice, tequila, and salt in a small bowl.

2. Make the ceviche: Combine the shrimp, pepper rings, radishes, cucumbers, red onion, cilantro, scallions, mint, and jalapeño in a large bowl. Add the marinade, gently toss to coat, then gently fold in the avocado. Chill in the refrigerator while you make the tortillas, stirring gently once or twice.

3. Make the tortillas: Preheat the oven to 400°F.

4. Arrange the tortillas on 2 rimmed baking sheets. Spray the tortillas lightly with the olive oil cooking spray, then bake until crisp and lightly golden, 7 to 8 minutes. Let cool about 5 minutes.

5. Serve the ceviche: Place a tortilla on 8 individual plates and mound some ceviche on each. Or, serve the ceviche in small bowls or cocktail glasses and offer the tortillas alongside.

Note: The ceviche is best if eaten within 30 minutes.

NUTRITIONAL INFORMATION (1 SERVING = 1 SCANT CUP, PLUS 1 TORTILLA) Calories 187, Total Fat 5.4 g 8%, Saturated Fat 0.8 g 4%, Trans Fat 0.0 g, Cholesterol 119.6 mg 40%, Sodium 923.4 mg 38%, Total Carb 18.9 g 6%, Dietary Fiber 4 g 16%, Sugars 2.2 g, Added Sugars 0 g, Protein 15.4 g 31%, Vitamin D 2.3 mcg 1%, Calcium 88.8 mg 9%, Iron 0.9 mg 5%, Potassium 387.6 mg 11%

NOOM CHEF'S TIP: HOW TO DICE AN AVOCADO *To easily dice an avocado, cut it in half and remove the pit, leaving the flesh in the peel. Using a small, sharp knife, make vertical cuts down through the flesh of each half to the peel, then make horizontal cuts also down through the flesh to the peel. Use a spoon to carefully scoop the diced avocado into the bowl, being sure to scoop down to the peel to avoid mashing the cubes.*

Crunchy Open-Faced Tuna Salad Sandwiches

¼ cup plain nonfat Greek yogurt

2 tablespoons light mayonnaise

Juice and zest of ½ small lemon (1 tablespoon juice and ½ teaspoon zest)

1½ teaspoons Dijon mustard

¼ teaspoon kosher salt

2 5-ounce cans chunk white tuna in water, well drained

¼ cup finely diced water chestnuts

1 large celery stalk, finely diced

1 medium carrot, finely shredded

2 tablespoons finely diced red onion

1 tablespoon finely diced pickled jalapeño (optional)

16 small butter lettuce leaves

1 large ripe tomato, thinly sliced into 8 rounds

8 slices thin whole-grain sandwich bread, toasted if desired

Serving sandwiches open faced is a great way to reduce the amount of bread you're eating and increase the amount of filling, as happens in this recipe with its serving size of two sandwiches. Look for thin, relatively small sandwich bread or pita about the size of a large tomato slice, and toast it first if you like a firmer base for your tuna salad.

SERVES 4 TOTAL TIME: 15 MINUTES

1. Make the tuna salad: In a medium bowl, whisk together the yogurt, mayonnaise, lemon juice and zest, mustard, and salt. Add the tuna, water chestnuts, celery, carrot, red onion, and jalapeño if using. Mix to combine well. You should have 2 cups of tuna salad.

2. Assemble and serve the sandwiches: Layer 2 lettuce leaves and 1 tomato slice on each of 8 bread slices. Top each tomato slice with ¼ cup of the tuna salad. Place 2 sandwiches on each of 4 plates and serve immediately.

NUTRITIONAL INFORMATION (1 SERVING = 2 OPEN-FACED SANDWICHES, WITH ½ CUP TUNA SALAD) Calories 199, Total Fat 4.4 g 7%, Saturated Fat 0.8 g 4%, Trans Fat 0.0 g, Cholesterol 17.3 mg 6%, Sodium 557.1 mg 23%, Total Carb 22.1 g 7%, Dietary Fiber 4.3 g 17%, Sugars 4.4 g, Added Sugars 0 g, Protein 17 g 34%, Vitamin D 0.0 mcg 0%, Calcium 128.6 mg 13%, Iron 2.1 mg 12%, Potassium 377.2 mg 11%

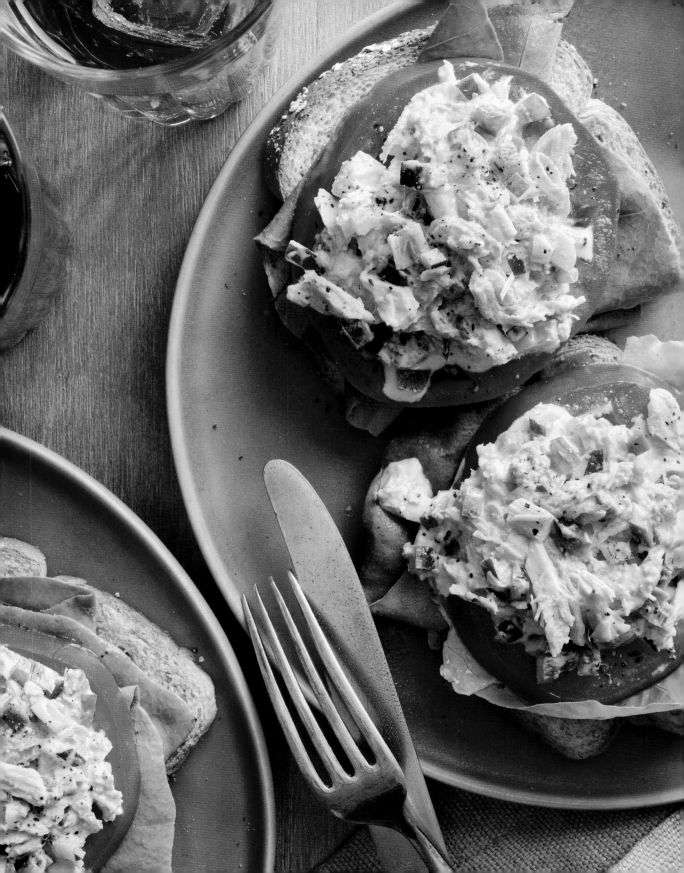

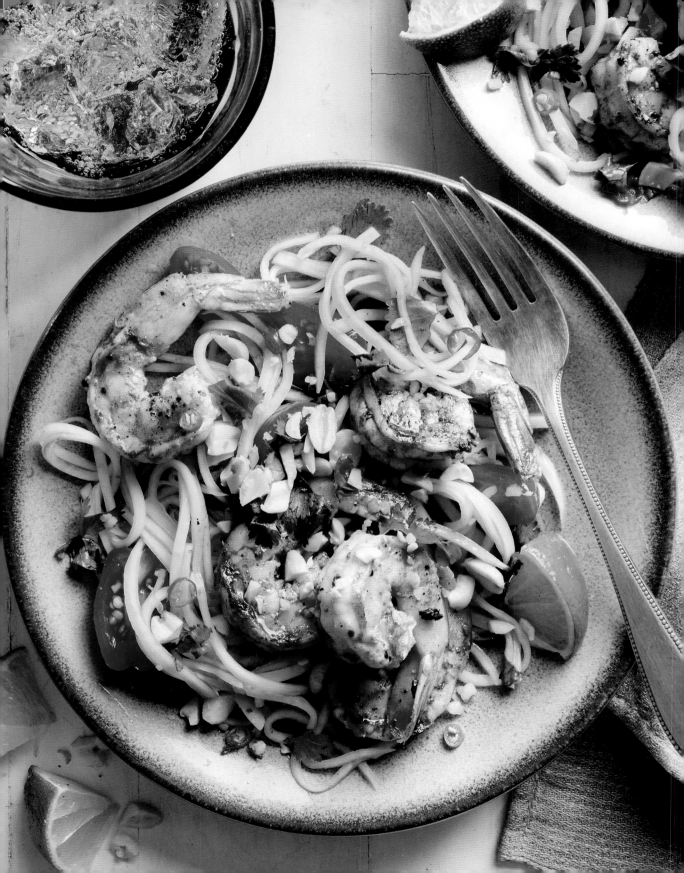

Grilled Shrimp & Papaya Salad

Use young green papayas rather than ripe orange ones for this recipe. Green papayas have a firm flesh that is not sweet yet, as it will be when ripened. The firmness here makes it easy to grate, and its mild flavor is a perfect backdrop for the spicy-sweet kick of this salad.

SERVES 4 TOTAL TIME: 30 MINUTES

FOR THE SHRIMP AND PAPAYA

1 small lime

1 tablespoon olive oil or grapeseed oil

¼ teaspoon kosher salt

¼ teaspoon cayenne or Thai (bird's-eye) chili flakes

1 pound large (20–30 count) shrimp, peeled and cleaned (thawed, if frozen)

1 large green papaya (about 2 pounds; see Note)

FOR THE DRESSING

4 garlic cloves

1 fresh Thai (bird's-eye) chili, thinly sliced (seeds removed for less heat)

2 tablespoons Thai or Vietnamese fish sauce

1½ tablespoons palm sugar or light brown sugar

½ teaspoon kosher salt

6 cherry tomatoes, halved

⅓ cup fresh cilantro leaves

2 tablespoons chopped roasted unsalted peanuts (or cashews)

1. Prepare the shrimp: Grate the zest from half the lime into a large bowl (reserve the lime).

2. Add the olive oil, salt, and cayenne. Then add the shrimp, toss to coat, and let marinate on the counter while you prepare the rest of the salad.

3. Prepare the papaya: Peel the papaya, then use a box grater or julienne peeler to shred the papaya into strands; you need about 4 cups.

4. Prepare the dressing and salad: Cut the reserved lime in half. Cut the unzested side into 4 wedges.

5. Juice the zested half and add the juice to a small bowl. Add the garlic, Thai chili, and fish sauce. Muddle or mash the chili and garlic to incorporate them into the dressing for more flavor (not necessary to pulverize).

6. Add the palm sugar and salt, then add the tomatoes and mash again lightly until the tomatoes soften and release some of their juices.

7. Grill the shrimp: If using wooden skewers, soak them in water for at least 15 minutes. Heat a grill to medium-hot or preheat a stovetop grill pan over medium-high heat.

8. Thread the shrimp onto the skewers, then grill until they turn bright pink, 1 to 2 minutes per side. Transfer to a plate.

9. Assemble and serve the salad: Add the grated papaya and the cilantro leaves to the tomato mixture and toss to combine.

continued on page 150

continued from page 149

10. Divide the salad among 4 bowls, then distribute the shrimp among the bowls and garnish each bowl with some peanuts. Serve the salads with lime wedges. Enjoy immediately.

Note: The recipe requires you to shred the papaya, but some grocery stores sell pre-shredded papaya. This salad can also be placed in a bowl and chilled for up to 4 hours, then served cold.

NUTRITIONAL INFORMATION (1 SERVING = 7 OR 8 SHRIMP, PLUS 1 CUP SALAD AND 2 TABLESPOONS DRESSING) Calories 231, Total Fat 6.8 g 11%, Saturated Fat 1.0 g 5%, Trans Fat 0.0 g, Cholesterol 142.9 mg 48%, Sodium 1644.8 mg 69%, Total Carb 26.6 g 9%, Dietary Fiber 3.7 g 15%, Sugars 17.9 g, Added Sugars 0 g, Protein 18.2 g 36%, Vitamin D 2.3 mcg 1%, Calcium 111.2 mg 11%, Iron 1.1 mg 6%, Potassium 573.7 mg 16%

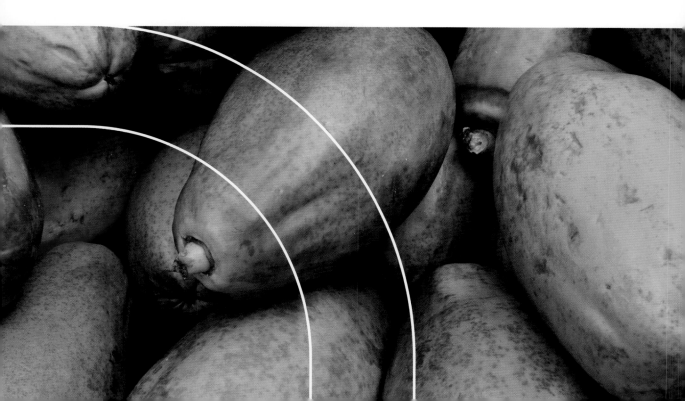

White Fish with Sweet Peppers

This mild fish transforms into a festive dinner when accompanied by a bright relish made from multicolored baby peppers.

FOR THE RELISH

1 tablespoon olive oil

2 garlic cloves, thinly sliced

6 tablespoons water

3 tablespoons sherry vinegar

1 teaspoon honey

2 teaspoons chopped fresh oregano (or ½ teaspoon dried)

¼ teaspoon kosher salt

8 multicolored baby peppers, seeded and thinly sliced into rings

1 medium orange

FOR THE FISH

4 6-ounce skin-on fish fillets (such as sea bass, cod, snapper), patted dry

½ teaspoon salt

4 teaspoons canola oil

2 tablespoons thinly sliced scallion greens

SERVES 4 TOTAL TIME: 20 MINUTES

1. Make the relish: Heat the olive oil in a small saucepan over medium-low heat. Add the garlic and cook until fragrant, about 2 minutes. Add the water, vinegar, honey, oregano, and salt. Bring to a boil and cook about 1 minute. Add the peppers and cook, stirring often, until they begin to soften but don't become mushy, about 5 minutes.

2. Transfer the pepper mixture to a bowl and set aside to cool for about 10 minutes.

3. Section the orange, then add the sections and any juice to the bowl with the pepper mixture.

4. Cook the fish: Season both sides of the fish fillets with the salt. Heat a medium (9- or 10-inch) skillet over medium-high heat.

5. Add 2 teaspoons of the oil, then use a heatproof pastry brush to spread the oil around the pan.

6. Add 2 of the fillets, skin side down, and cook, pressing down on the fish with a fish spatula, until the skin is crisped and deep golden, 4 to 5 minutes. Flip and cook until the fish is opaque and flaky, 2 to 3 more minutes.

7. Repeat with the remaining 2 teaspoons oil and 2 remaining fish fillets.

continued on page 152

continued from page 151

8. Serve the fish: Arrange the fish fillets on a large serving platter, then spoon the relish over them and sprinkle with the scallion greens. Serve.

NUTRITIONAL INFORMATION (1 SERVING = 1 FISH FILLET, PLUS ⅓ CUP RELISH) Calories 262, Total Fat 11 g 17%, Saturated Fat 1.6 g 8%, Trans Fat 0.1 g, Cholesterol 58.1 mg 19%, Sodium 378.2 mg 16%, Total Carb 12.8 g 4%, Dietary Fiber 2.4 g 10%, Sugars 10 g, Added Sugars 0 g, Protein 27.2 g 55%, Vitamin D 320.4 mcg 80%, Calcium 45.5 mg 5%, Iron 1.0 mg 6%, Potassium 571.4 mg 16%

NOOM CHEF'S TIP: SEEDING PEPPERS *Sweet peppers are usually used without their seeds. The seeds from hot peppers make a dish quite a lot hotter, but seeds from sweet peppers are tasteless and add nothing to a dish. It's easy to cut the seeds and pith from the flesh of large sweet peppers, but to do so from very small—so-called baby—peppers, cut off the tops and then scrape out the seeds with a small spoon (such as a ¼ teaspoon measuring spoon) before slicing or chopping. And remember: when removing the seeds from hot peppers, use gloves and avoid touching your eyes.*

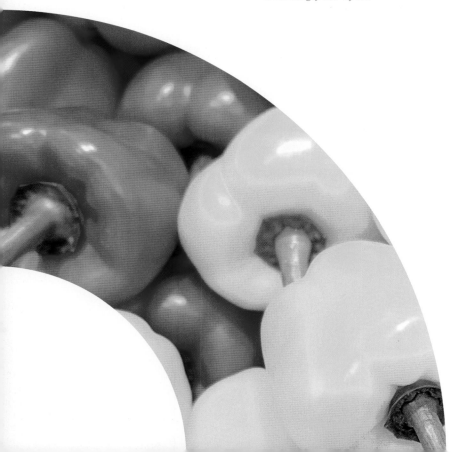

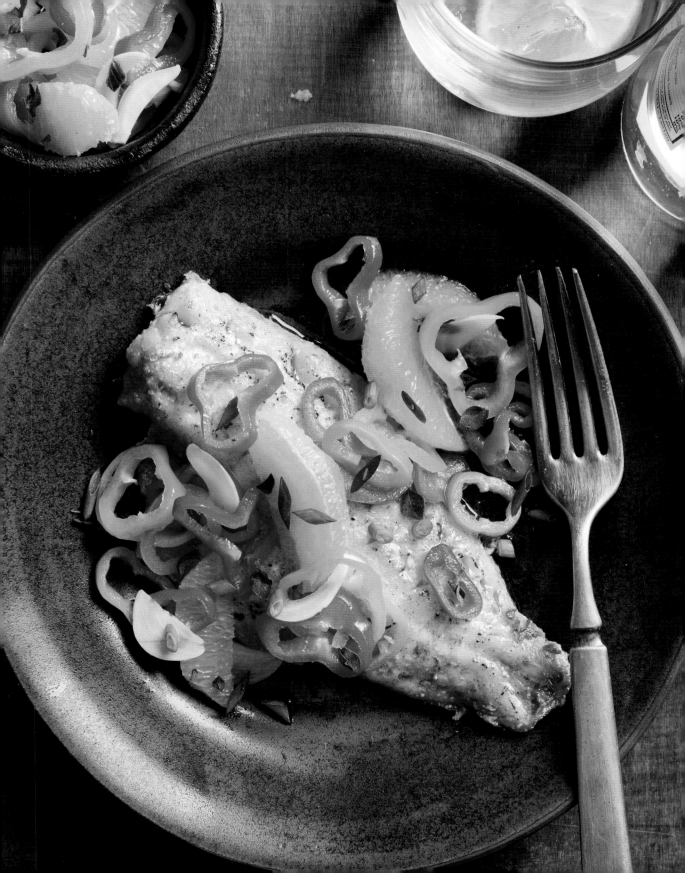

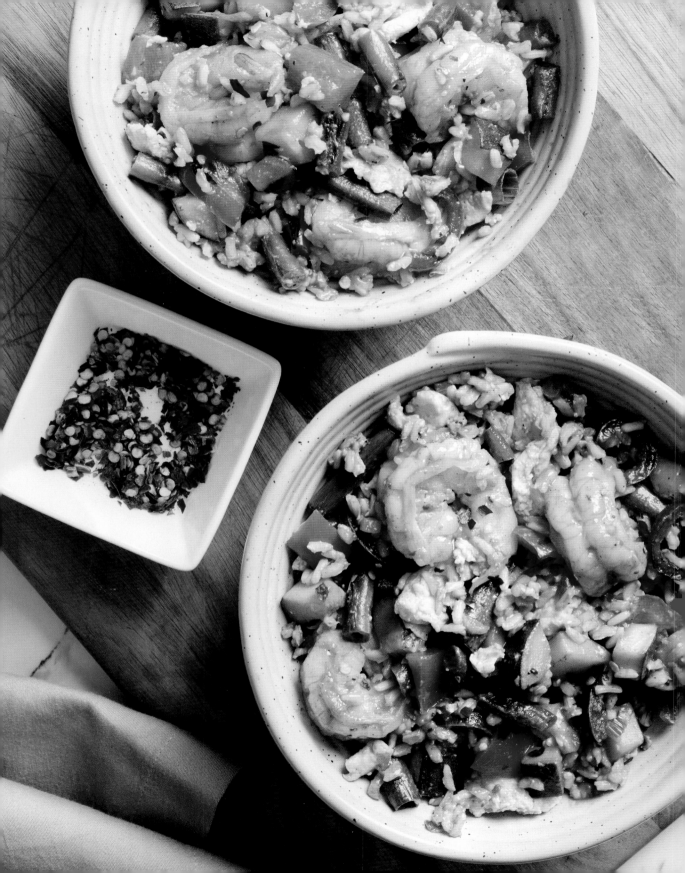

Shrimp & Veggie Fried Rice

If you've been waiting for a reason to break out that wok you've had stored in a cupboard, this is your chance. If you don't have a wok, though, you can still easily make this crispy-savory stir-fry in a deep-fry pan or skillet with high sides. Make sure you give yourself plenty of room for mixing all the ingredients!

SERVES 4 TOTAL TIME: 45 MINUTES

1. Make the sauce: Combine the soy sauce, chicken broth, oyster sauce, and sesame oil in a small bowl.

2. Cook the rice according to the package instructions.

3. Marinate the shrimp: Toss the shrimp with the sesame oil and salt.

4. Cook the separate elements for the stir-fry: Heat 2 teaspoons of the oil in a large (12-inch) skillet or wok over medium-high heat.

5. Add the beaten eggs and cook, stirring, until just scrambled, 1 to 2 minutes. Transfer to a plate.

6. Add 2 more teaspoons of the oil to the skillet, then add the shrimp and cook, stirring, until the shrimp just turns pink, about 1 minute. Transfer to a plate.

7. Add the remaining 2 teaspoons oil to the skillet, then add the scallion whites, ginger, and garlic, and cook, stirring, until fragrant, about 2 minutes. Add the bell pepper, zucchini, green beans, jalapeño, and broth. Cover the skillet and cook, stirring midway, 3 to 4 minutes.

8. Build the stir-fry and serve: Add the rice to the skillet and stir to incorporate. Add the sauce and cook, stirring, until warmed through and the rice has absorbed the sauce, 2 to 3 minutes.

9. Stir in the shrimp and the scrambled eggs, and cook to warm through, 1 to 2 minutes more.

10. Stir in the scallion greens, then divide the stir-fry among 4 plates and serve hot.

FOR THE SAUCE

3 tablespoons soy sauce

¼ cup low-sodium chicken broth or water

1 tablespoon oyster sauce

1 tablespoon toasted sesame oil

FOR THE RICE

¾ cup long-grain brown rice

FOR THE SHRIMP

12 ounces fresh large shrimp, peeled and cleaned, tails removed (or 1¼ pounds frozen prepared shrimp, thawed)

1 teaspoon toasted sesame oil

¼ teaspoon salt

FOR THE STIR-FRY

2 tablespoons peanut oil

4 large eggs, lightly beaten

4 scallions, thinly sliced, green and white parts kept separate

1 2-inch piece of fresh ginger, very finely minced

5 garlic cloves, minced

1 large red or yellow bell pepper, cut into ¼-inch pieces

1 large zucchini, cut into ¼-inch cubes

4 ounces green beans, trimmed and cut into ¼-inch pieces

½ jalapeño, seeded and thinly sliced

¼ cup chicken broth, plus more as needed

NUTRITIONAL INFORMATION (1 SERVING = 2 CUPS) Calories 425, Total Fat 18.6 g 29%, Saturated Fat 3.8 g 19%, Trans Fat 0.1 g, Cholesterol 293 mg 98%, Sodium 1596.3 mg 67%, Total Carb 40.1 g 13%, Dietary Fiber 4.5 g 18%, Sugars 5.7 g, Added Sugars 0 g, Protein 25.2 g 50%, Vitamin D 42.7 mcg 11%, Calcium 134.6 mg 13%, Iron 3.1 mg 17%, Potassium 736.7 mg 21%

Zucchini-Wrapped Pesto Fish Fillets

Thinly sliced zucchini is the perfect veggie to encase tender fish and a brightly flavored pesto. Fresh basil and Parmesan cheese add a ton of flavor. This comes together in just a few minutes of active time, but it looks and tastes like it took hours. So easy! Dinner is a wrap.

FOR THE PESTO

1 cup packed fresh basil leaves

¼ cup finely grated Parmigiano-Reggiano cheese

3 tablespoons walnuts

2 tablespoons water

1 tablespoon fresh lemon juice

1 teaspoon finely grated lemon zest

1 garlic clove

¼ teaspoon kosher salt

¼ teaspoon freshly ground black pepper

FOR THE FISH

4 5-ounce white fish fillets (such as sea bass, cod, tilapia), patted dry

¾ teaspoon kosher salt

¾ teaspoon freshly ground black pepper

2 small zucchini (about 8 ounces total)

1 tablespoon olive oil

1½ cups cherry tomatoes

Fresh basil leaves, for garnish

SERVES 4   TOTAL TIME: 40 MINUTES

1. Make the pesto: Combine the basil, cheese, walnuts, water, lemon juice and zest, garlic, salt, and pepper in the small bowl of a food processor and process, stopping the processor and scraping down the sides of the bowl if necessary, until you have a unified, slightly grainy paste, 15 to 20 seconds.

2. Wrap and bake the fish: Preheat the oven to 400°F.

3. Line a rimmed baking sheet or 9-by-13-inch baking dish with parchment. Arrange the fish fillets on the baking sheet and season well with ¼ teaspoon each of the salt and pepper.

4. Spread 1½ tablespoons of the pesto on each fillet.

5. Use a vegetable peeler to peel wide strips from the zucchini. Wrap 3 or 4 zucchini strips around each fillet, tucking the ends underneath.

6. Brush the zucchini strips with ½ tablespoon of the oil.

7. Arrange the tomatoes all around and in between the fish fillets, and drizzle them with the olive oil. Season the tomatoes and zucchini strips with the remaining ½ teaspoon each salt and pepper.

8. Bake until the tomatoes are shriveled and slightly charred, the zucchini is soft, and the fish is cooked through, 18 to 20 minutes. (If your wrapped fillets haven't browned on top, remove them from the oven, turn on the broiler, and broil just until the zucchini is golden in spots, 1 to 2 minutes).

9. Serve the fish wraps: Carefully use a spatula to lift the fish fillets onto 4 individual plates, then spoon the tomatoes around each. Serve at once.

NUTRITIONAL INFORMATION (1 SERVING = 1 FISH WRAP, WITH 1½ TABLESPOONS PESTO) Calories 250, Total Fat 11.6 g 18%, Saturated Fat 3.1 g 15%, Trans Fat 0.0 g, Cholesterol 64.4 mg 21%, Sodium 516.6 mg 22%, Total Carb 6 g 2%, Dietary Fiber 2 g 8%, Sugars 3.1 g, Added Sugars 0 g, Protein 30.8 g 62%, Vitamin D 320.4 mcg 80%, Calcium 131 mg 13%, Iron 1.3 mg 7%, Potassium 714.8 mg 20%

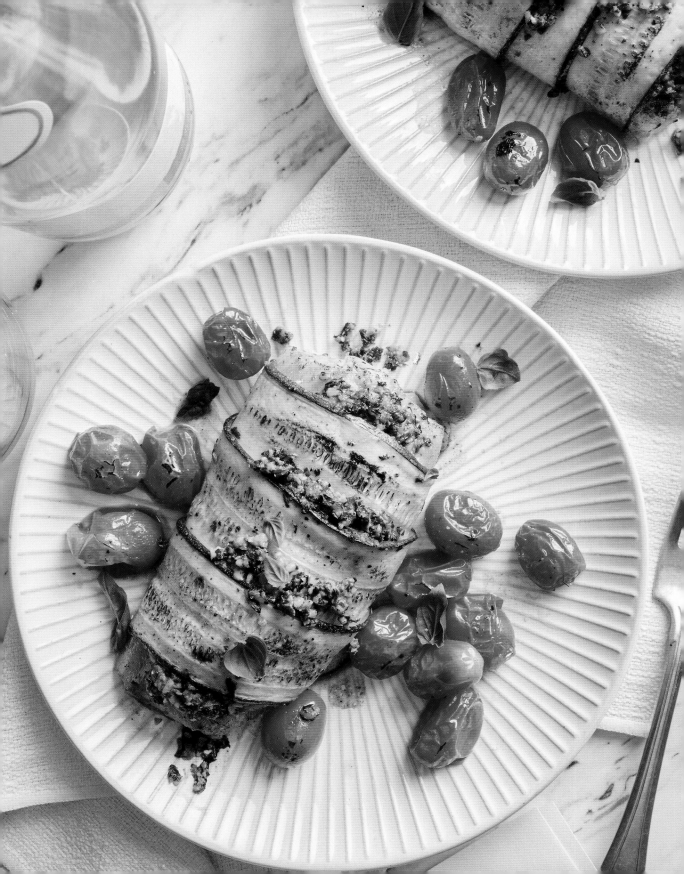

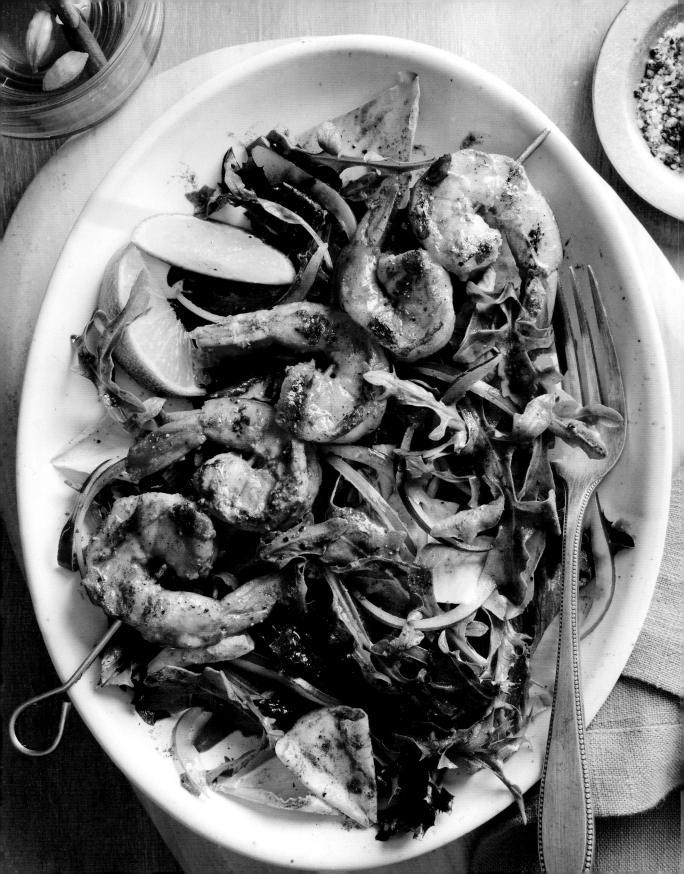

Tandoori Shrimp

⅓ cup plain nonfat Greek yogurt

Grated zest and juice from
1 lime (2 teaspoons juice and
1 teaspoon zest)

2 garlic cloves, finely minced

2 teaspoons finely minced fresh
ginger

1 teaspoon garam masala

½ teaspoon kosher salt

½ teaspoon sweet paprika

⅛ to ¼ teaspoon cayenne

1 pound jumbo shrimp
(16–20 count), shelled and
cleaned, patted dry

FOR THE DRESSING

1 teaspoon garam masala

2 tablespoons olive oil

2 tablespoons fresh lime juice

1 teaspoon honey

Pinch of kosher salt

FOR SERVING

8 cups assorted mixed greens
(arugula, butter lettuce, etc.)

¼ cup thinly sliced red onion

Kosher salt

Toss fresh greens with an herby, toasty vinaigrette and top with these Indian-inspired shrimp skewers for a tasty meal full of flavor and nutrients.

SERVES 4   TOTAL TIME: 1 HOUR (INCLUDING MARINATING)

1. If using wooden skewers, arrange the skewers in a rimmed dish and cover with cold water to soak for 30 minutes.

2. Marinate the shrimp: In a large bowl, whisk together the yogurt, lime juice and zest, garlic, ginger, garam masala, salt, paprika, and cayenne. Add the shrimp, stir to coat with the marinade, and let sit on the counter for 15 to 30 minutes.

3. Make the dressing: While the shrimp is marinating, warm the garam masala in a small saucepan over medium heat until fragrant, 2 to 3 minutes. Add the olive oil and cook 1 more minute, then transfer to a bowl and let cool for 5 minutes.

4. Whisk in the lime juice, honey, and salt.

5. Grill the shrimp: Heat a grill to very hot or preheat a stovetop grill pan over high heat. Spray the grill with nonstick cooking spray.

6. Thread 4 to 5 shrimp onto each skewer. Grill the shrimp (close the grill, if using an outdoor grill) until lightly charred on each side, flipping once, until just cooked through, 3 to 4 minutes per side. The yogurt marinade will harden slightly on the exterior.

7. Place the skewers on a plate and cover lightly to keep warm.

continued on page 160

continued from page 159

8. Assemble the dish and serve: Arrange the greens and red onion in a large bowl, add the remaining dressing, toss, then transfer to a large serving platter. Top with the shrimp skewers (or remove the shrimp from the skewers and place on top of the greens). Season to taste with salt and serve hot or at room temperature.

NUTRITIONAL INFORMATION (1 SERVING = 4 TO 5 SHRIMP, PLUS 2 CUPS SALAD) Calories 188, Total Fat 8.1 g 13%, Saturated Fat 1.1 g 6%, Trans Fat 0.1 g, Cholesterol 143.6 mg 48%, Sodium 923.7 mg 38%, Total Carb 9.8 g 3%, Dietary Fiber 1.4 g 6%, Sugars 2.7 g, Added Sugars 0 g, Protein 18.8 g 38%, Vitamin D 2.3 mcg 1%, Calcium 148 mg 15%, Iron 3.2 mg 18%, Potassium 193.1 mg 6%

NOOM CHEF'S TIP: USING SKEWERS *Skewers are handy kitchen items if you like to grill foods like shrimp, veggie chunks, or tofu cubes. If you use wooden skewers, you need to soak them in cold water for about 15 minutes before grilling; this keeps them from burning. If you use metal skewers, be careful—they can get hot!*

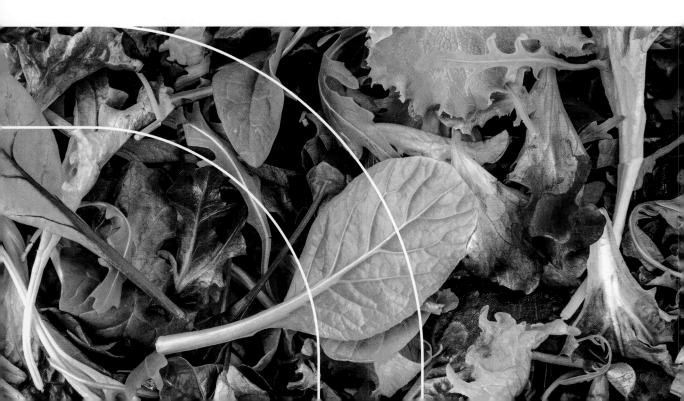

Seafood Stew with Crispy Toasts

This delicious seafood stew will feed a crowd or a large family, but you can easily cut the recipe in half to serve 4. If there are leftovers, know that they will keep in the refrigerator only for about one day, but alternatively you could freeze them for up to about 2 weeks.

FOR THE STEW BASE

3 tablespoons olive oil

1 medium fennel bulb, trimmed, quartered, cored, and sliced

1 medium onion, chopped

3 medium carrots, chopped

3 large celery stalks, halved lengthwise and diced

3 garlic cloves, minced

1 teaspoon kosher salt

½ teaspoon freshly ground black pepper

1 tablespoon harissa paste, plus more to taste

½ cup dry white wine

6 ripe medium tomatoes (about 2 pounds), cored and diced (or a 28-ounce can diced tomatoes)

2 tablespoons chopped preserved lemon (or 1 tablespoon finely chopped fresh lemon, rind included)

6 cups low-sodium chicken broth (or fish stock)

1 tablespoon fresh lemon juice

FOR THE TOASTS

16 ¼-inch baguette slices

Olive oil

1 garlic clove, halved

FOR FINISHING THE STEW AND SERVING

8 ounces calamari, cut into rings

8 ounces large shrimp, shelled and cleaned

12 ounces white fish fillet (such as cod or snapper), cut into 1-inch pieces

1 tablespoon fresh lemon juice

¼ teaspoon chopped fresh parsley, plus more for garnish

Kosher salt and freshly ground black pepper

SERVES 8 TOTAL TIME: 90 MINUTES

1. Prepare the stew base: Heat the olive oil in a large (6-quart) heavy-bottomed pot over medium-high heat. Add the fennel, onion, carrots, and celery and cook, stirring, until the vegetables begin to soften, about 5 minutes.

2. Add the garlic, salt, pepper, and harissa and cook, stirring, about 1 minute. Add the wine and cook until most of the liquid evaporates, about 5 minutes.

3. Add the tomatoes, preserved lemon, broth, and lemon juice. Bring to a boil, then reduce the heat to medium-low. Cover and simmer, stirring occasionally, until the vegetables absorb some of the liquid and are tender, about 30 minutes.

continued on page 163

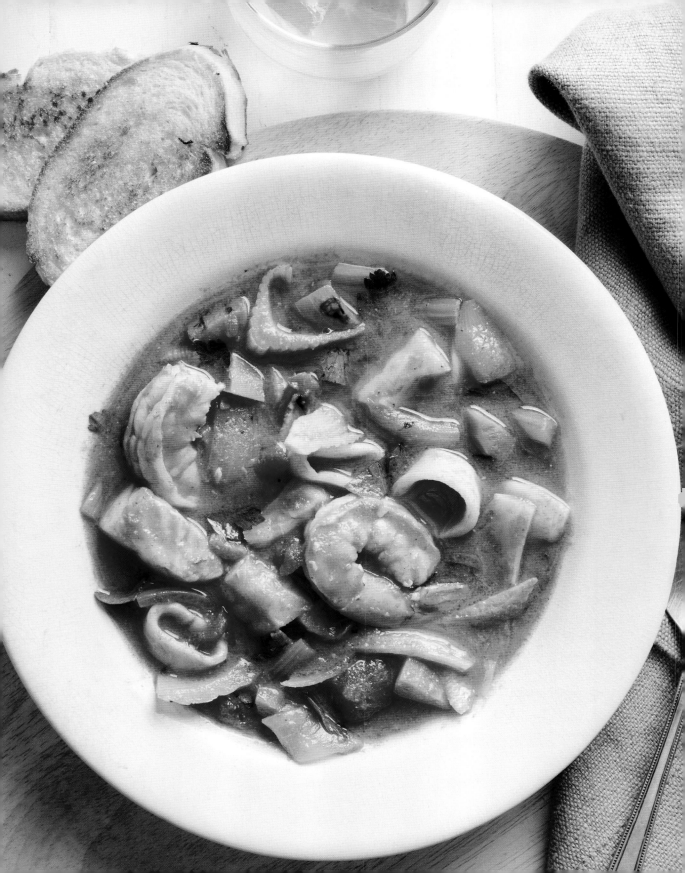

continued from page 161

4. Make the toasts: Ten minutes before serving, set a rack in the top third of the oven and preheat the broiler. Arrange the bread slices in a large baking pan (a ribbed or grill pan will give the bread nice grill marks). Very lightly brush the top of each bread slice with a little olive oil. Broil the bread slices until the tops are lightly golden and toasted, making sure not to let them burn, about 30 seconds.

5. Rub the toasted sides of each bread slice with the cut sides of the halved garlic.

6. Finish and serve the stew: Five minutes before serving, gently stir the calamari, shrimp, and fish into the stew.

7. Simmer, uncovered, until the seafood is opaque and just cooked through, 5 to 6 minutes.

8. Stir in the lemon juice and most of the parsley, season with salt and pepper, then divide the stew among 8 bowls and garnish with the remaining parsley.

9. Serve with 2 toasts per person, on the side.

NUTRITIONAL INFORMATION (1 SERVING = 1¼ CUPS, PLUS 2 BAGUETTE SLICES) Calories 317, Total Fat 10.2 g 16%, Saturated Fat 1.5 g 8%, Trans Fat 0.0 g, Cholesterol 125.1 mg 42%, Sodium 711.3 mg 30%, Total Carb 30.3 g 10%, Dietary Fiber 4 g 16%, Sugars 7.6 g, Added Sugars 0 g, Protein 23.9 g 48%, Vitamin D 203.8 mcg 51%, Calcium 92.4 mg 9%, Iron 1.5 mg 8%, Potassium 839.6 mg 24%

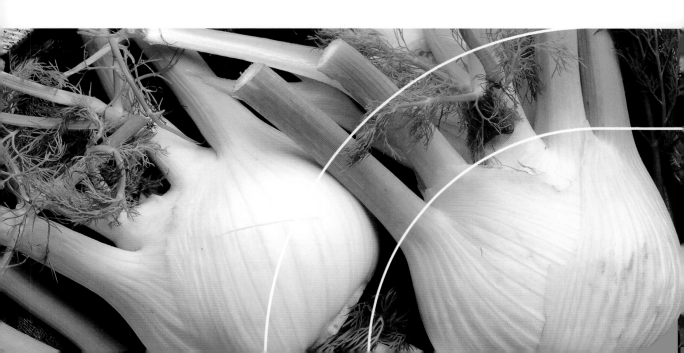

Salmon & Cucumber Hand Rolls

8 ounces sushi-grade salmon fillet (see Note), skin, pin bones, and any gray parts removed

1 tablespoon light mayonnaise

1 tablespoon low-sodium soy sauce, plus more for serving

2 teaspoons unseasoned rice wine vinegar (or rice vinegar)

1½ teaspoons toasted sesame oil

1 teaspoon wasabi powder or wasabi paste, plus more for serving

¼ teaspoon kosher salt

1 small cucumber (about 4 ounces), peeled, seeds removed, very finely diced

¼ cup chopped scallion greens, plus more for garnish

1 tablespoon drained and chopped pickled ginger, plus more for serving

¾ cup cooked brown rice (or Scallion-y Cauliflower & Brown Rice, page 204)

6 nori sheets

1½ teaspoons toasted sesame seeds

Pickled ginger, wasabi paste, and/or low-sodium soy sauce, for serving (optional)

Be sure to purchase sushi-grade salmon for this recipe, and keep it chilled until right before you prepare the meal. These hand rolls are fun to make and eat—no trip to a sushi restaurant required.

SERVES 2 TOTAL TIME: 20 MINUTES

1. Prepare the filling: Finely dice the salmon and add it to a medium bowl; chill until ready to use.

2. When ready to serve, whisk together in a small bowl the mayonnaise, 1 tablespoon soy sauce, the vinegar, sesame oil, 1 teaspoon wasabi, and the salt. Fold the seasoning into the salmon, then gently fold in the cucumber, scallion greens, and 1 tablespoon pickled ginger.

3. Assemble the hand rolls: See photos and instructions on page 27.

4. Sprinkle the top of each cone with ¼ teaspoon sesame seeds and some scallions.

5. Serve the hand rolls: Arrange the hand rolls on a platter or on 2 individual serving plates. Serve immediately, with additional pickled ginger, wasabi, and soy sauce, if desired.

Note: Consuming raw or undercooked seafood may increase the risk of foodborne illness. Be sure to use sushi-grade salmon here, and prepare this dish on the day you purchase the fish.

NUTRITIONAL INFORMATION (1 SERVING = 3 HAND ROLLS) Calories 368, Total Fat 14.5 g 22%, Saturated Fat 2.1 g 11%, Trans Fat 0.1 g, Cholesterol 62.7 mg 21%, Sodium 954.2 mg 40%, Total Carb 29.7 g 10%, Dietary Fiber 5.4 g 22%, Sugars 4.1 g, Added Sugars 0 g, Protein 30.4 g 61%, Vitamin D 500.1 mcg 125%, Calcium 71.1 mg 7%, Iron 2.1 mg 12%, Potassium 596.3 mg 17%

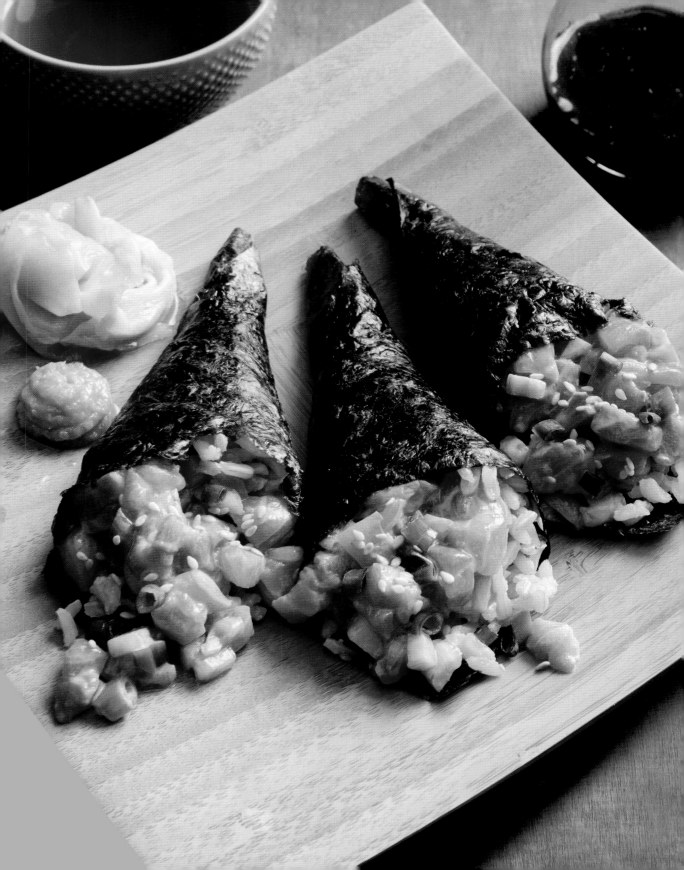

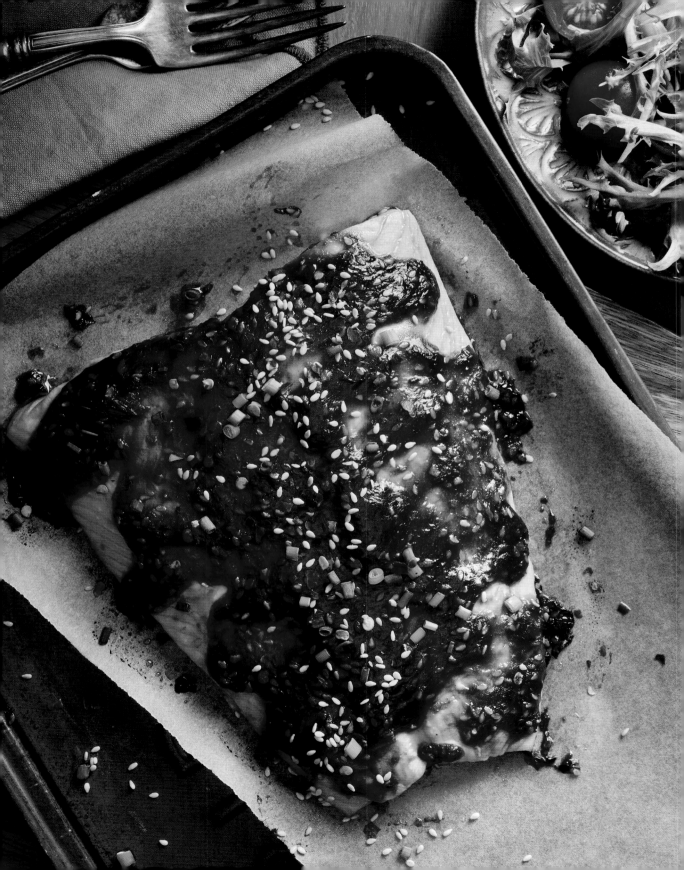

Teriyaki Salmon

Serve this Asian-inspired salmon with a simple salad of mixed greens for a light dinner, or pair it with any of the side salads in this book (pages 84–107). You could also add the Scallion-y Cauliflower & Brown Rice (page 204) or the Herbed Whole-Grain Couscous (page 221) for a more substantial meal.

FOR THE SAUCE

¼ cup fresh orange juice

2 tablespoons light soy sauce

1½ teaspoons rice vinegar

2 tablespoons water

2 teaspoon cornstarch

2 tablespoons finely grated fresh ginger (or 1 teaspoon ground ginger)

2 garlic cloves, finely minced

1½ teaspoons toasted sesame oil

¼ teaspoon red pepper flakes

1 1-pound salmon fillet, skin removed and fish patted dry

2 teaspoons sesame seeds

FOR SERVING

1 teaspoon sesame seeds

1 tablespoon chopped fresh chives

Red pepper flakes (optional)

SERVES 4 TOTAL TIME: 25 TO 30 MINUTES

1. Preheat the oven to 400° F.

2. Make the sauce: Add the orange juice, soy sauce, rice vinegar, and water to a small saucepan, then whisk in the cornstarch until dissolved. Add the ginger, garlic, sesame oil, and red pepper flakes.

3. Place the saucepan over medium heat and bring the liquid to a low boil, then reduce the heat to low and simmer until the sauce thickens, 1 to 2 minutes. Remove the saucepan from the heat and cool the sauce to room temperature. This should take 10 to 15 minutes.

4. Bake the salmon: Line a baking sheet or baking dish with parchment and place the salmon on it. Brush the fillet with the sauce, then sprinkle with the sesame seeds and bake until just cooked through, 10 to 20 minutes.

5. Serve the salmon: Gently transfer the salmon to a serving platter. Cut the fillet into 4 equal pieces. Garnish the servings with the sesame seeds and sprinkle with the chives. If desired, top with additional red pepper flakes.

NUTRITIONAL INFORMATION (1 SERVING = ¼ OF THE SALMON) Calories 284, Total Fat 17.8 g 27%, Saturated Fat 3.8 g 19%, Trans Fat 0.0 g, Cholesterol 62.4 mg 21%, Sodium 401.7 mg 17%, Total Carb 5.7 g 2%, Dietary Fiber 0.4 g 1%, Sugars 2.4 g, Added Sugars 0 g, Protein 24.1 g 48%, Vitamin D 500.1 mcg 125%, Calcium 16.8 mg 2%, Iron 0.8 mg 4%, Potassium 458.4 mg 13%

Vegetarian

It's just not true that dinner is incomplete without meat. When you leave meat off the plate, you make room for a whole new world of vegetables, grains, beans, nuts, seeds, and fruit. You may find yourself eating a rainbow of foods, with more variety than you ever did before! This chapter will give you plenty of great ideas, and will dispel any notions that vegetables are boring.

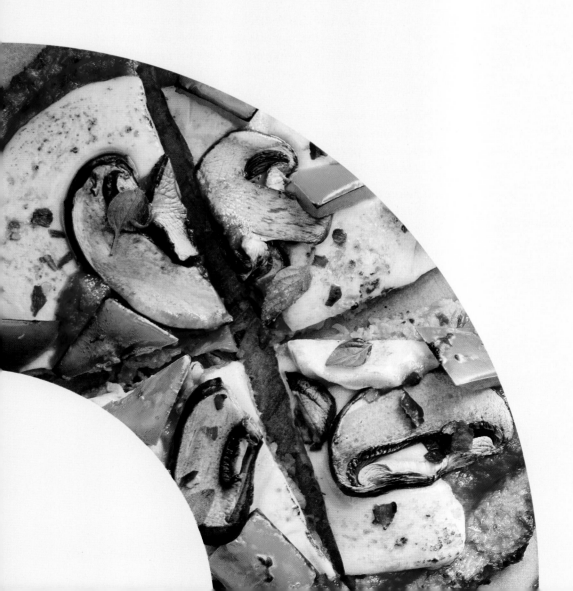

Cauliflower Pizza Crust

There is nothing wrong with regular pizza crust, but sometimes you might want something lighter and less rich in carbs. Cauliflower pizza crust to the rescue! This recipe makes single-serving crusts that taste great but are delicate. Keep your toppings on the dry side, and if you add veggies, sauté them first to eliminate the moisture, or they could make your cauliflower crust soggy.

FOR THE CRUST

1 large head cauliflower (or 1¾ pounds florets)

¾ cup finely shredded Parmigiano-Reggiano cheese

⅓ cup shredded mozzarella cheese

2 large eggs, lightly beaten

1 teaspoon garlic powder

1 teaspoon onion powder

1 teaspoon kosher salt

½ teaspoon freshly ground black pepper

SUGGESTED TOPPINGS

Pizza sauce (look for sugar-free), low-sugar BBQ sauce, shredded mozzarella cheese, sliced mushrooms, sliced red onions, diced bell peppers, sliced olives, shredded cooked chicken, crumbled cooked turkey sausage, turkey pepperoni, chopped fresh basil, dried oregano.

SERVES 8 TOTAL TIME: 50 MINUTES

1. Prep and cook the cauliflower: Use a knife to remove the leaves and core from the cauliflower. Break it into florets.

2. Working in 2 batches, pulse the cauliflower florets in a food processor until uniform large grains form, about 45 seconds per batch. You should have about 8 cups finely chopped cauliflower.

3. Place the cauliflower in a large (12-inch) nonstick skillet with a lid. Cover and cook over medium heat, uncovering often and stirring to prevent the cauliflower from sticking to the skillet, until mostly tender and dry, 10 to 11 minutes. Uncover and let cool somewhat, about 5 minutes.

4. Line a rimmed baking sheet with a clean kitchen towel, then spread the cauliflower on the towel. Top with another towel and press firmly all over to absorb any excess liquid.

5. Prepare the dough and bake the crusts: Preheat the oven to 450°F. Line 2 or 3 baking sheets with parchment.

6. Add the cauliflower to a large bowl, then add the Parmigiano-Reggiano and mozzarella cheeses, the eggs, garlic and onion powders, salt, and pepper. Stir until well incorporated.

7. Using a ½ cup measure, scoop up 8 packed portions of the cauliflower dough. Turn these out onto the baking sheets. Using your hands, press each piece into a 6-inch round, leaving at least 1 inch between crusts. You should be able to fit 3 or 4 crusts on each sheet.

8. Bake until the dough dries and the edges and top are browned, about 15 minutes. Remove from the oven (leaving the oven on), let cool for 5 minutes, then use a metal spatula to carefully release and flip the crusts on the baking sheets. Bake until further dried, about an additional 5 minutes.

continued on page 172

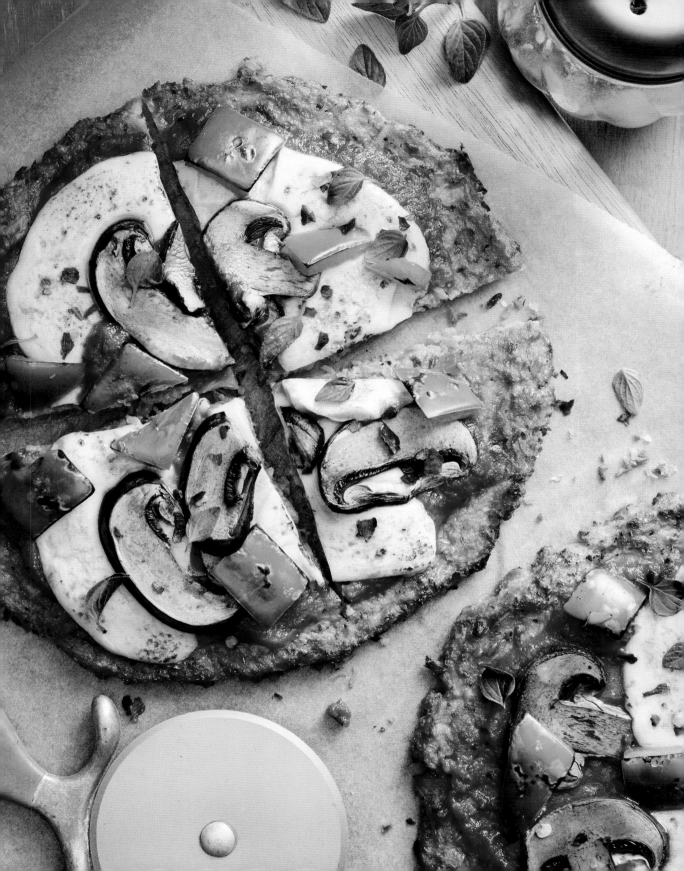

continued from page 170

9. Top, warm, and serve the pizzas: Add any toppings you would like to the crusts, or let everyone add their own toppings. Return the crusts to the oven long enough to warm the toppings, melt any added cheese, and so on. Serve the individual pizzas hot.

Note: If you won't be serving all 8 crusts at the same time, you can freeze the baked crusts. Let them cool completely, then layer them in a large zippered freezer bag with sheets of parchment or waxed paper in between the crusts. To reheat, remove the crusts you need and put them on a baking sheet. Bake in a 450°F oven for 5 minutes, then add your desired toppings. Place back in the oven and bake until the sauce is hot and the cheese is melted, 6 to 8 more minutes.

NUTRITIONAL INFORMATION (1 SERVING = 1 PIZZA CRUST WITHOUT TOPPINGS) Calories 113, Total Fat 6.1 g 9%, Saturated Fat 3.7 g 18%, Trans Fat 0.0 g, Cholesterol 62.1 mg 21%, Sodium 363.2 mg 15%, Total Carb 6.2 g 2%, Dietary Fiber 2.2 g 9%, Sugars 2.2 g, Added Sugars 0 g, Protein 9.5 g 19%, Vitamin D 11.4 mcg 3%, Calcium 221.7 mg 22%, Iron 0.8 mg 4%, Potassium 349 mg 10%

NOOM CHEF'S TIP *You can top this pizza crust with any of your favorite pizza toppings, keeping in mind that the crust is pretty delicate and might get soggy with too many toppings. Aim for approximately 2 to 3 tablespoons of sauce, 2 to 3 tablespoons of cheese, and about ¼ cup total of toppings per individual crust—the more veggies the better!*

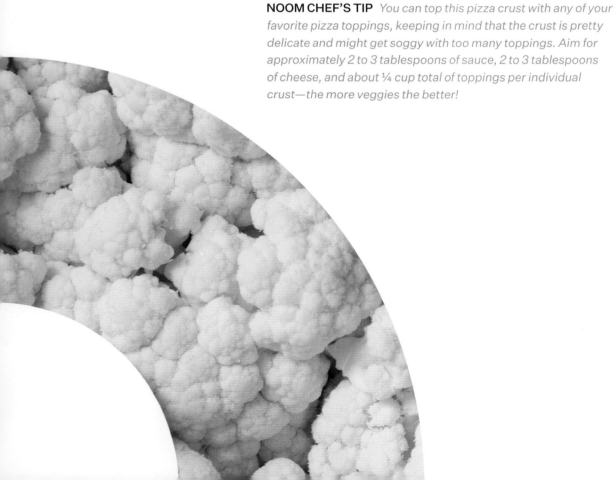

Spiced Eggplant Steaks

Eggplant has the perfect texture for a veggie steak, and it absorbs all the flavors of the herbs, spices, and sauce you add to it. Topped with a juicy veggie relish and creamy tahini sauce, this recipe is totally plant based and so loaded with flavor that you won't even miss the beef.

FOR THE EGGPLANT

2 medium eggplants, trimmed and halved lengthwise

4 teaspoons olive oil

Kosher salt and freshly ground black pepper

½ teaspoon ground turmeric

½ teaspoon ground cumin

½ teaspoon sweet paprika

Pinch of cayenne (optional)

FOR THE RELISH

5 Persian cucumbers, trimmed and diced

¼ cup sliced onion

¼ cup fresh mint leaves, chopped

¼ cup fresh parsley leaves, chopped

2 tablespoons fresh lemon juice

1 teaspoon finely grated lemon zest

½ teaspoon salt

FOR THE TAHINI SAUCE

3 tablespoons tahini

3 tablespoons water

3 tablespoons fresh lemon juice

½ teaspoon finely grated lemon zest

¼ teaspoon kosher salt, plus more for seasoning

½ cup pomegranate seeds

Freshly ground black pepper

SERVES 4   TOTAL TIME: 1 HOUR

1. Bake the eggplant: Preheat the oven to 400°F. Line a baking sheet with parchment.

2. Use a sharp knife to lightly score the cut sides of the eggplant halves in a crosshatch pattern, then brush each on the cut side with 1 teaspoon of the olive oil. Season to taste with salt and pepper.

3. Arrange the eggplant halves, cut sides down, on the baking sheet and bake until the eggplant has softened in spots but is firm in others, about 25 minutes.

4. While the eggplant is baking, combine the remaining 3 teaspoons olive oil with the turmeric, cumin, paprika, and cayenne, if using, in a small bowl. Flip the eggplant halves, then brush the cut sides with the spiced oil and return to the oven and continue to bake until the tops are deeply golden and the eggplant is tender, 15 to 20 minutes more.

continued on page 175

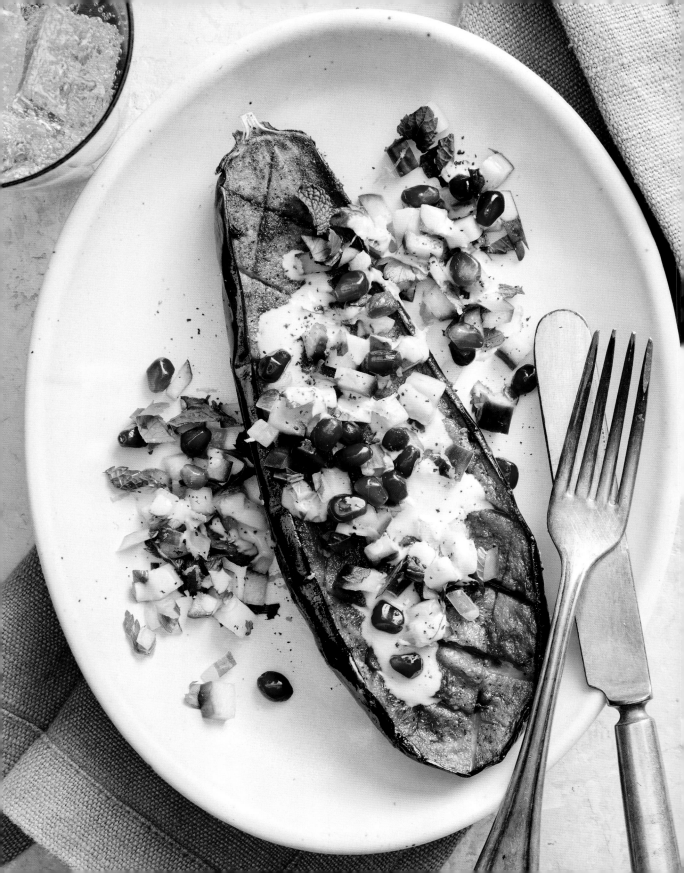

continued from page 173

5. Make the relish: While the eggplant is roasting, combine the cucumbers, onion, mint, parsley, lemon juice and zest, and salt in a bowl. Cover and chill in the refrigerator until ready to use.

6. Make the tahini sauce: Whisk the tahini, water, lemon juice and zest, and salt in a small bowl.

7. Serve the eggplant: Arrange each baked eggplant half on an individual plate, then top each with about ¾ cup of the relish. Drizzle with about 2 tablespoons of the tahini sauce, sprinkle with 2 tablespoons of the pomegranate seeds, and season to taste with more salt and pepper.

NUTRITIONAL INFORMATION (1 SERVING = 1 EGGPLANT HALF, ¾ CUP RELISH, 2 TABLESPOONS TAHINI SAUCE, AND 2 TABLESPOONS POMEGRANATE SEEDS) Calories 214, Total Fat 11.7 g 18%, Saturated Fat 1.6 g 8%, Trans Fat 0.0 g, Cholesterol 0.0 mg 0%, Sodium 500.2 mg 21%, Total Carb 27.5 g 9%, Dietary Fiber 10.9 g 44%, Sugars 11.7 g, Added Sugars 0 g, Protein 5.9 g 12%, Vitamin D 0.0 mcg 0%, Calcium 102.6 mg 10%, Iron 2.5 mg 14%, Potassium 883.9 mg 25%

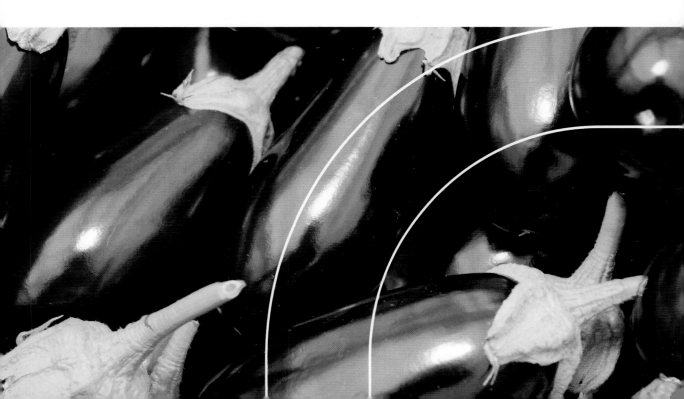

Charred Cabbage Wedges with Chimichurri

We at Noom love eggs, and we think they're a great protein choice for every meal—not just breakfast! Here's a twist on breakfast. The charred cabbage wedges stand in for toast, and the zippy chimichurri—a spicy garlic and herb sauce from Argentina—jazzes up the eggs. This is a meal your family and friends will rave about for days, no matter what time of day you decide to serve it! (Or keep it all to yourself!)

FOR THE CHIMICHURRI

⅓ cup finely chopped fresh parsley

3 tablespoons finely minced shallot

3 tablespoons water

2 tablespoons olive oil

1½ tablespoons red wine vinegar

2 garlic cloves, finely minced

1 small fresh red chile, seeded and finely minced

½ teaspoon kosher salt

½ teaspoon dried oregano

¼ teaspoon finely ground black pepper

FOR THE CABBAGE AND EGGS

1 large (about 4 pounds) head green cabbage, cored and cut into 8 thin wedges

2 tablespoons olive oil

½ teaspoon kosher salt, plus more for seasoning

½ teaspoon freshly ground black pepper, plus more for seasoning

Olive oil cooking spray

8 large eggs

SERVES 4   TOTAL TIME: 35 MINUTES

1. Make the chimichurri: In a medium bowl, combine the parsley, shallot, water, olive oil, vinegar, garlic, chile, salt, oregano, and black pepper; cover and refrigerate until ready to use.

2. Make the cabbage: Preheat the oven to 425°F.

3. Brush both sides of the cabbage wedges with the olive oil, then arrange on a rimmed baking sheet. Sprinkle the tops with the salt and pepper and roast until the cabbage is slightly softened and the edges are charred, 25 to 30 minutes, flipping the wedges about halfway through cooking.

4. Make the eggs: Heat a small (8-inch) skillet over medium heat. Spray with cooking spray, then cook 2 eggs, sunny side up, until the whites are opaque but the yolks are still runny, 2 to 3 minutes. Transfer to a plate and cover lightly to keep warm.

5. Repeat 3 times more with the remaining 6 eggs and using more cooking spray.

6. Serve the dish: Arrange 2 cabbage wedges on each of 4 plates, then arrange a fried egg on each cabbage wedge. Dollop about 1 tablespoon of the chimichurri on each egg, and season to taste with additional salt and pepper.

NUTRITIONAL INFORMATION (1 SERVING = 2 CABBAGE WEDGES, 2 EGGS, 2 TABLESPOONS CHIMICHURRI) Calories 356, Total Fat 23.4 g 36%, Saturated Fat 5.1 g 26%, Trans Fat 0.1 g, Cholesterol 372 mg 124%, Sodium 574 mg 24%, Total Carb 22 g 7%, Dietary Fiber 8.6 g 34%, Sugars 11.4 g, Added Sugars 0 g, Protein 17.2 g 34%, Vitamin D 82 mcg 20%, Calcium 200.6 mg 20%, Iron 4 mg 22%, Potassium 762.3 mg 22%

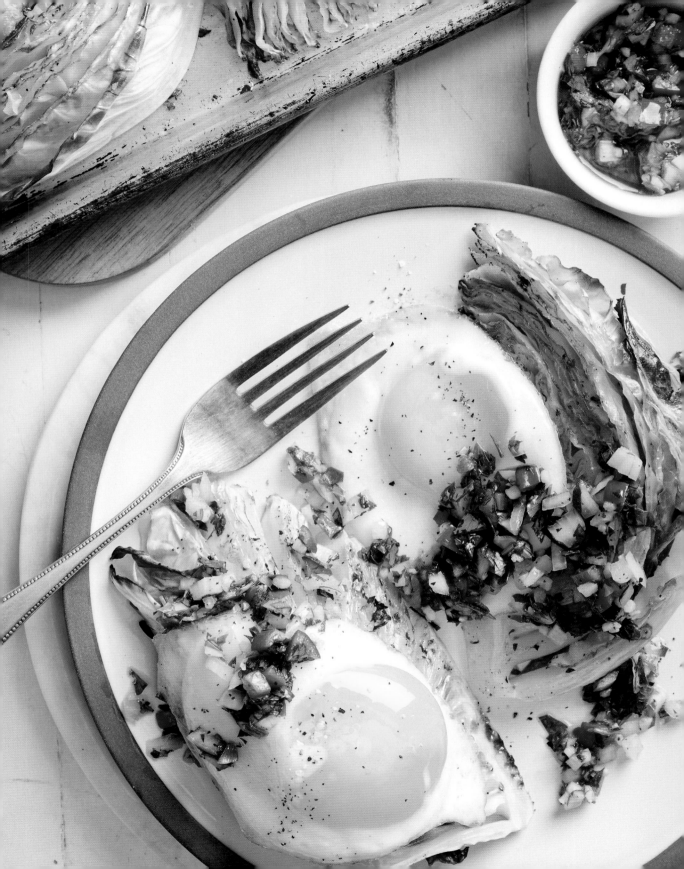

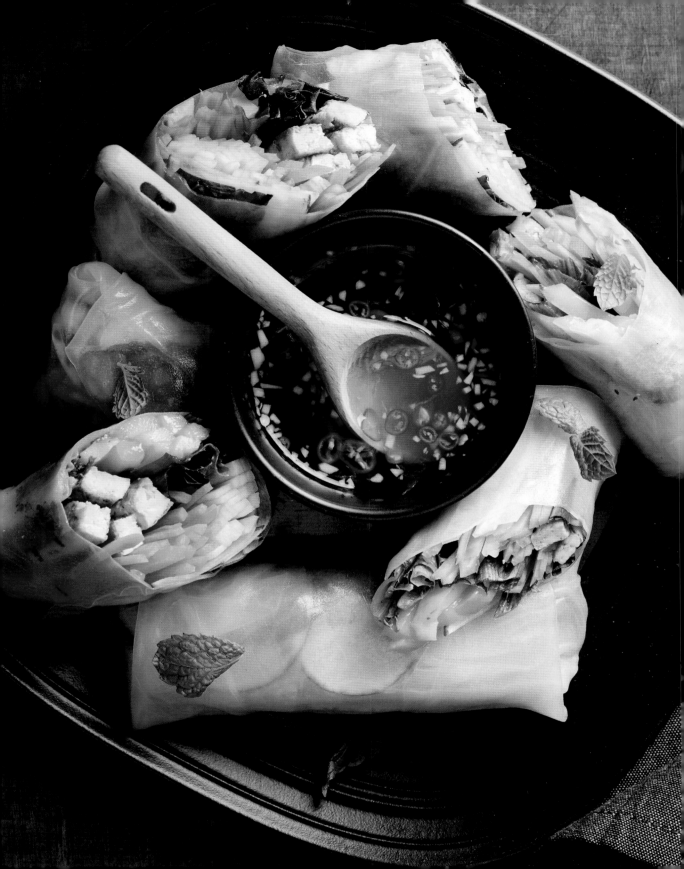

Tofu & Mango Summer Rolls

It can take some practice to wrap a summer roll without tearing the delicate rice-paper wrapper. See our photos here, demonstrating how to do it. If you mess up the first few, that's okay—practice makes perfect!

FOR THE DIPPING SAUCE

2 small limes

1 tablespoon fish sauce

1 tablespoon water

2 teaspoons light brown sugar or palm sugar

2 teaspoons unseasoned rice wine vinegar

1 teaspoon sliced Thai (bird's-eye) chili (or any small hot chili)

1 garlic clove, very finely minced

FOR THE ROLLS

½ 14-ounce package extra-firm tofu

2 tablespoons low-sodium soy sauce

8 8-inch round rice wrappers

16 large fresh basil leaves

2 small radishes, very thinly sliced

4 to 6 red-leaf lettuce leaves, rinsed and patted dry, center stems removed, leafy parts cut into 3-by-1-inch rectangles

2 small carrots, julienned into 3-inch strips

2 small Persian cucumbers, peeled and julienned into 3-inch strips

½ firm, ripe mango, peeled and julienned into 3-inch strips

16 to 24 small fresh mint leaves

SERVES 4   TOTAL TIME: 1 HOUR 15 MINUTES

1. Make the sauce: Finely zest the limes into a medium bowl and set the zest aside. Halve and juice the limes (about ¼ cup juice) into a small bowl. Add the fish sauce, water, brown sugar, vinegar, chili, and garlic, and stir to dissolve the brown sugar, about 30 seconds.

2. Sear and slice the tofu: Pat the tofu dry, then cut into ¼-inch slices (4 or 5 slices).

3. Preheat a large (12-inch), dry (no oil or spray) nonstick skillet over medium-high heat. Place the tofu slices in the pan and press down on them for 10 seconds, then let them fry for about 3 minutes; the tofu will begin to release water.

4. After about 4 minutes, the undersides will be browned and crisp; flip the tofu and repeat the process until both sides are browned and crisp, another 3 to 4 minutes.

5. Cool and cut into thin strips. Add the strips to the bowl of lime zest and toss to coat. Sprinkle with the soy sauce and toss to coat again. Wash and dry the skillet.

6. Assemble the summer rolls: For photos and instructions, see page 27.

7. Serve the summer rolls: Place 2 rolls each on 4 individual plates and serve immediately with the dipping sauce.

Note: To store the rolls for a couple of hours, cover them on all sides with dampened clean kitchen towels.

NUTRITIONAL INFORMATION (1 SERVING = 2 ROLLS, PLUS 2 TABLESPOONS DIPPING SAUCE) Calories 160, Total Fat 01.8 g 2%, Saturated Fat 0.4 g 2%, Trans Fat 0.0 g, Cholesterol 0.0 mg 0%, Sodium 920.6 mg 38%, Total Carb 30.8 g 10%, Dietary Fiber 2.6 g 10%, Sugars 11.6 g, Added Sugars 0 g, Protein 6.6 g 14%, Vitamin D 0.0 mcg 0%, Calcium 63.2 mg 6%, Iron 01.6 mg 8%, Potassium 409.6 mg 12%

Sweet Potato Shepherd's Pie

A traditional shepherd's pie has a top crust of pillowy mashed potatoes over a meaty lamb stew, but this version places nutritious sweet potatoes over a rich mushroom filling This adds color and some extra vegetables, but keeps all the warm, cozy flavors that make the pie a household favorite! Serve with one of our bright side salads to complement the savory quality of this dish.

FOR THE TOPPING

1 jumbo or 2 medium sweet potatoes (about 1½ pounds total), peeled and cubed

½ head large cauliflower, trimmed and florets separated

2 tablespoons plain unsweetened almond milk

1 tablespoon unsalted butter

1 teaspoon salt

¼ teaspoon freshly ground black pepper

1 large egg

FOR THE FILLING

2½ pounds fresh mushroom caps (mix of portobello, baby bella, and button)

2 tablespoons olive oil

1 medium onion, finely diced

1 celery stalk, finely diced

1 medium carrot, finely diced

4 garlic cloves, thinly sliced

2 tablespoons tomato paste

2 teaspoons Worcestershire sauce

1 teaspoon kosher salt, plus more for seasoning

½ teaspoon freshly ground black pepper, plus more for seasoning

¼ teaspoon cayenne

3 tablespoons cornstarch

3 tablespoons water

¼ cup chopped fresh parsley, plus more for garnish

2 teaspoons fresh thyme leaves, plus more for garnish

Sweet paprika

SERVES 6   TOTAL TIME: 1 HOUR 35 MINUTES

1. Make the topping: Combine the sweet potatoes and cauliflower florets in a microwave-safe dish, add ½ inch of water, seal tightly with plastic wrap, and microwave on high until the sweet potatoes and cauliflower are tender, about 8 minutes. Uncover, drain, and cool for about 10 minutes.

2. To the bowl of a food processor add the sweet potatoes and cauliflower, then add the almond milk, butter, salt, and pepper. Process until smooth, 1 to 2 minutes, stopping to scrape the sides as needed. Add the egg and process until smooth again, about 10 more seconds. Transfer the topping to a medium bowl. Wipe out the bowl of the food processor.

3. Chop the mushrooms: Working in batches, add the mushrooms to the food processor and pulse to chop into ¼-inch pieces, 25 to 30 pulses per batch. You should have about 12 cups of chopped mushrooms.

4. Make the filling: Heat a large (12-inch) skillet over medium-high heat. Add 1 tablespoon of the olive oil, then add the onion, celery, carrot, and garlic and cook, stirring often, until the vegetables soften and the onion is translucent, 7 to 8 minutes.

5. Add the remaining tablespoon oil. Working in batches, add the mushrooms, adding more mushrooms as those in the pan begin to wilt, about 8 minutes, stirring as you go.

continued on page 182

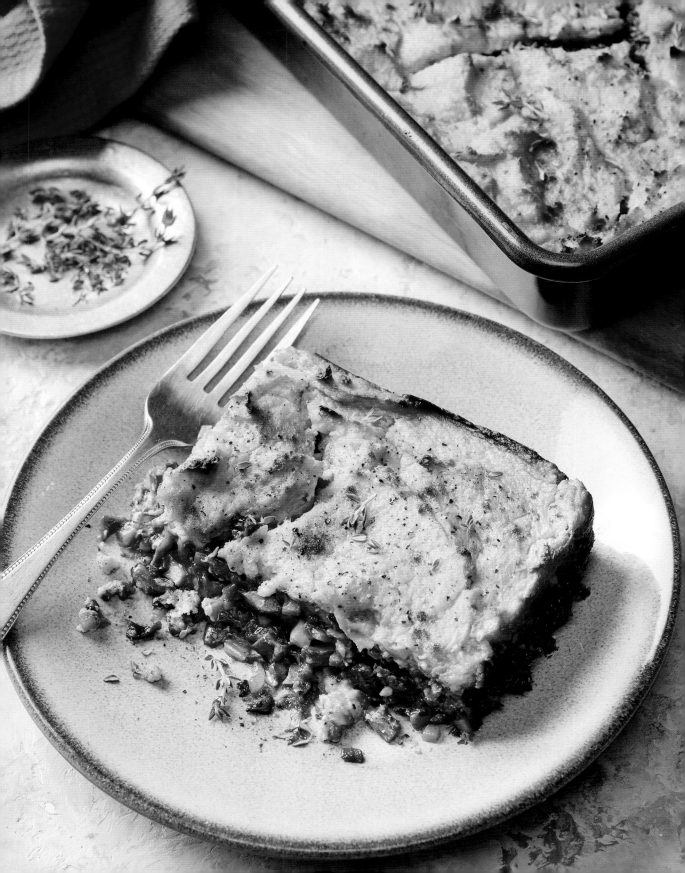

continued from page 180

6. Add the tomato paste, Worcestershire sauce, teaspoon salt, and ½ teaspoon pepper, then the cayenne. Cook, stirring well, for 1 to 2 minutes.

7. In a small bowl, whisk together the cornstarch and water, then whisk the cornstarch mixture into the mushrooms. Cook, stirring thoroughly, until slightly thickened, about 1 minute. Remove from the heat and stir in the parsley and thyme.

8. Assemble the pie: Preheat the oven to 400°F. Spray the bottom and sides of a 9-inch square baking dish with cooking spray.

9. Spread the mushroom mixture in the dish until smooth. Using a measuring tablespoon, dot the sweet potato mixture over the mushrooms and spread it evenly across the top.

10. Bake and serve: Bake the pie until the top is firm and golden tipped, and the filling is slightly bubbling up, 45 to 50 minutes. Let the pie rest for 15 minutes to settle, then cut into 6 rectangles and serve on 6 individual plates. Sprinkle each with additional parsley and thyme, and add a dash of paprika. Serve.

NUTRITIONAL INFORMATION (1 SERVING = 3-INCH SQUARE) Calories 258, Total Fat 8.2 g 13%, Saturated Fat 2.3 g 11%, Trans Fat 0.1 g, Cholesterol 36.1 mg 12%, Sodium 826.5 mg 34%, Total Carb 40.3 g 13%, Dietary Fiber 7.4 g 30%, Sugars 11.7 g, Added Sugars 0 g, Protein 10.3 g 21%, Vitamin D 21.5 mcg 5%, Calcium 92.3 mg 9%, Iron 3 mg 17%, Potassium 1290.3 mg 37%

Coconut-Crusted Piri Piri Tofu

 This recipe uses tangy-spicy piri piri sauce, a type of hot pepper sauce from Africa, to enliven flavor-crusted tofu cubes. Topped with summertime succotash, a corn-based vegetable mixture that (in this recipe) also contains peppers and zucchini, this is a great dish for late summer, when all those wonderful veggies are at their peak. Use extra-firm tofu for the best texture.

SERVES 4 TOTAL TIME: 45 MINUTES

FOR THE TOFU

2 13-to-14-ounce blocks extra-firm tofu

1 large egg

2 teaspoons piri piri sauce

1 teaspoon kosher salt

3 tablespoons white whole wheat or rice flour

½ teaspoon smoked paprika

½ cup panko or other bread crumbs

½ cup unsweetened shredded coconut

Olive oil cooking spray

FOR THE SUCCOTASH

1 tablespoon vegetable oil

2 garlic cloves, thinly sliced

1 medium zucchini, finely diced

2 cups frozen corn kernels, thawed and drained

1 red bell pepper, cored, seeded, and finely diced

1 scallion (green and white parts), thinly sliced

2 tablespoons water

1 tablespoon unsalted butter

½ teaspoon kosher salt, plus more for seasoning

1. Prepare the tofu: Preheat the oven to 400°F. Line a baking sheet with parchment. Set the oven rack in the middle position.

2. Arrange the tofu between 2 sets of paper towels atop a plate and place a matching plate on top; weight down with a heavy can for 30 minutes to drain excess water from the tofu (or use a tofu press, if you have one).

3. Cut each tofu block in half horizontally.

4. Prepare the dip and breading: Whisk the egg in a shallow medium bowl along with 1 teaspoon of the piri piri sauce and ¼ teaspoon of the salt.

5. Combine the flour, ¼ teaspoon of the paprika, and another ¼ teaspoon of the salt in a medium bowl.

6. Combine the panko, coconut, and remaining ¼ teaspoon paprika in another bowl.

7. Bread the tofu: Dip each tofu slice in the flour, then in the egg, letting any excess egg drip off. Press the pieces into the panko-coconut mixture, pressing firmly on all sides to help the crumbs adhere. Arrange on the baking sheet.

8. Spray the tofu slices with the olive oil cooking spray and season both sides lightly with the remaining ½ teaspoon salt. Bake until slices are crispy, 20 to 25 minutes.

9. Remove the tofu slices from the oven and slice each piece into 6 strips (total of 24 pieces).

continued on page 185

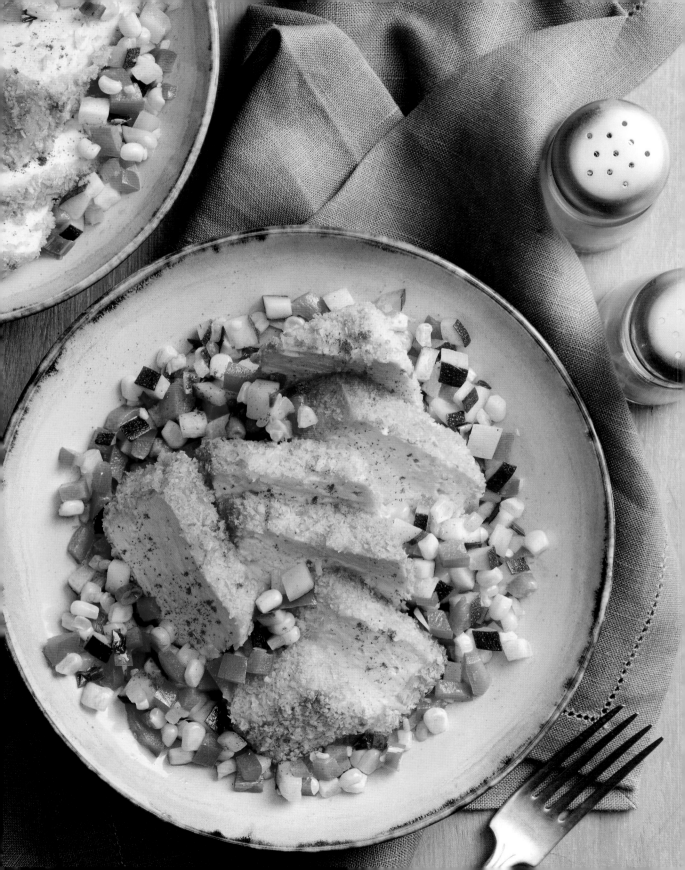

continued from page 183

10. Make the succotash: In a large (12-inch) skillet, heat the oil over medium-low heat. Add the garlic and cook until fragrant, 2 minutes. Add the zucchini, corn, bell pepper, scallion, and water. Raise the heat to medium, cover, and cook until all the vegetables are softened, about 5 minutes. Stir in the butter, add the remaining teaspoon piri piri sauce, and sprinkle with the salt, adding more to taste.

11. Serve: Divide the succotash among 4 bowls and top each bowl with 6 tofu strips. Serve warm.

NUTRITIONAL INFORMATION (1 SERVING = 1 CUP SUCCOTASH AND ½ BLOCK TOFU)
Calories 402, Total Fat 21.9 g 34%, Saturated Fat 12.2 g 61%, Trans Fat 0.2 g, Cholesterol 54.1 mg 18%, Sodium 854.5 mg 36%, Total Carb 33.4 g 11%, Dietary Fiber 7.4 g 30%, Sugars 7.3 g, Added Sugars 0 g, Protein 20.4 g 41%, Vitamin D 12.4 mcg 3%, Calcium 85.5 mg 9%, Iron 4.5 mg 25%, Potassium 857.3 mg 24%

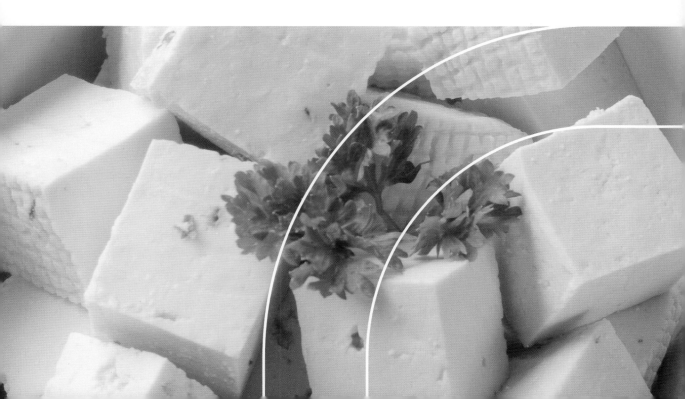

Broccoli & Orzo Risotto

3 cups vegetable broth

10 ounces fresh broccoli, finely chopped

1 tablespoon olive oil

½ cup finely minced shallots

3 garlic cloves, minced

1 cup orzo pasta

½ cup dry white wine

2 tablespoons chopped fresh basil, plus more for serving

½ cup finely grated Parmigiano Reggiano cheese, plus more for serving

1 teaspoon unsalted butter

¼ teaspoon salt, plus more for seasoning

Pinch of grated nutmeg

Freshly ground black pepper

Traditionally, the Italian dish risotto is made with arborio rice, a short grain that requires extended cooking and stirring. It's delicious, but time-consuming. This lighter version is faster, less calorically dense, and tastes just as decadent!

SERVES 4 TOTAL TIME: 30 MINUTES

1. Prepare the broth: In a medium saucepan, bring the broth to a low boil over medium-high heat. Reduce the heat to low, cover. and keep warm.

2. Steam the broccoli: Place the broccoli in a microwave-safe dish, add about ½ cup water, cover, and microwave on high until the broccoli turns bright green and stems are crisp-tender, about 2 minutes. Drain.

3. Sauté the shallots and orzo: Heat the olive oil in a medium saucepan over medium heat. Add the shallots and cook, stirring frequently, until fragrant and slightly translucent, 2 minutes. Add the garlic and cook, stirring constantly, 1 more minute.

4. Add the orzo and stir until coated and shiny, then add the wine and cook, stirring, until mostly evaporated, 1 to 2 minutes.

5. Make the risotto: Add the warm broth, ½ cup at a time, stirring constantly while cooking, waiting until each broth addition is fully absorbed by the orzo before adding more (3 to 4 minutes between additions). As the orzo cooks, it will release its starch and become creamy.

6. Cook the risotto for 14 to 15 minutes, adding about 2½ cups of the broth; only add the remaining ½ cup broth if the risotto looks dry or stiff. Taste the pasta. It should be firm to the bite but not hard in the center.

7. Finish and serve the risotto: Stir the broccoli into the risotto, then add the basil, Parmigiano-Reggiano, butter, salt, and nutmeg. Continue to cook, stirring, until just warmed through, 1 to 2 minutes. Season to taste with additional salt, if desired.

8. Divide the risotto among 4 bowls and garnish with additional basil and cheese, and grind some fresh pepper on top. Serve hot.

NUTRITIONAL INFORMATION (1 SERVING = 1 CUP) Calories 398, Total Fat 11.6 g 18%, Saturated Fat 5.3 g 26%, Trans Fat 0.2 g, Cholesterol 20 mg 7%, Sodium 685.6 mg 29%, Total Carb 56 g 19%, Dietary Fiber 5.3 g 21%, Sugars 5.9 g, Added Sugars 0 g, Protein 14.2 g 28%, Vitamin D 2.1 mcg 1%, Calcium 216.1 mg 22%, Iron 6.2 mg 35%, Potassium 326.7 mg 9%

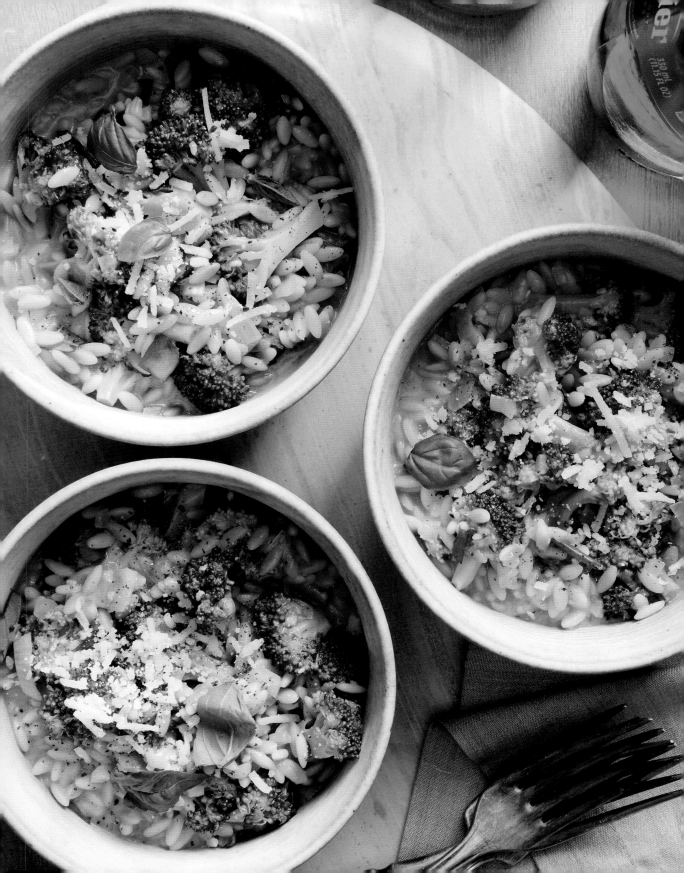

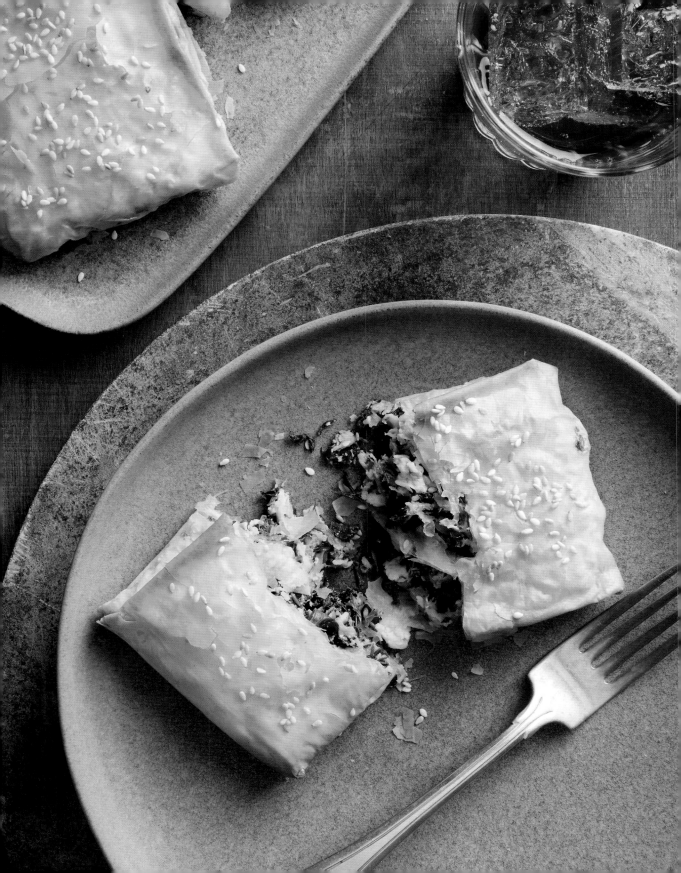

Spinach & Feta "Hot Pockets"

These DIY "hot pockets" are really more like Greek spanakopita, a wrapping of phyllo dough around a spinach and feta cheese filling. Phyllo (same as filo) is like puff pastry, but it is made with oil instead of butter. It bakes into a crispy crust of many thin layers, and it's easy to work with. Even if things get a little messy, the phyllo will still be irresistibly delicious, and you'll have an excuse to make it again for more practice.

FOR THE FILLING

1 tablespoon olive oil

1 medium zucchini, grated

¾ teaspoon kosher salt

1 pound frozen chopped spinach, thawed and drained

½ cup crumbled feta cheese

1 large egg, lightly beaten

3 tablespoons chopped fresh dill

3 tablespoons finely chopped fresh parsley

1 tablespoon minced garlic

1 teaspoon finely grated lemon zest

1 teaspoon chopped fresh oregano (or ½ teaspoon dried)

¼ teaspoon freshly ground black pepper

FOR MAKING THE POCKETS

12 9-by-14-inch sheets phyllo dough

Olive oil cooking spray

2 teaspoons sesame seeds

SERVES 4   TOTAL TIME: 50 MINUTES

1. Prepare the filling: Heat the olive oil in a medium nonstick saucepan over medium heat. Add the zucchini and ¼ teaspoon of the salt and cook, stirring, until the zucchini reduces by half its size and loses some of its moisture, about 6 minutes. Transfer the zucchini to a large bowl and set aside.

2. Spread the spinach in a line lengthwise across a clean cotton kitchen towel. Roll up the towel and twist to squeeze out as much excess liquid as possible.

3. Add the spinach to the zucchini in the bowl. Then stir in the feta, egg, dill, parsley, garlic, lemon zest, oregano, remaining ½ teaspoon salt, and pepper. Mix well to thoroughly combine. You should have a generous 2 cups of filling.

4. Assemble the pockets: Preheat the oven to 400°F. Line a baking sheet with parchment.

5. Unfold and arrange 1 sheet of phyllo on a large, clean work surface, with the short (9-inch) side closest to you, keeping the stack of remaining filo under a slightly damp, clean kitchen towel, to keep it from drying out.

6. Spray the phyllo sheet with the olive oil cooking spray for 5 seconds, covering the surface. Stack 2 more sheets of phyllo directly on top.

7. Measure out a generous ½ cup of the filling and spread it on the lower third of the sheet, leaving a 2-inch border along the bottom and sides. Fold the bottom length of phyllo up and over the filling, then fold the sides in, and fold up and over into a roughly 6-by-2-inch rectangle. Fold again, then arrange, seam side down, on the baking sheet.

continued on page 190

continued from page 189

8. Repeat this process 3 more times with the remaining phyllo to make 3 more stacks of 3 sheets each, with filling added and then folded to make a total of 4 pockets.

9. Spray the tops of the pockets with the cooking spray and sprinkle each with ½ teaspoon of the sesame seeds.

10. Bake and serve the pockets: Place the baking sheet with the pockets in the hot oven and bake until the pockets are golden and crisp, about 20 minutes. Serve hot.

Note: Alternatively, once cooled, the pockets can be wrapped in foil and frozen individually. They can then be thawed, unwrapped, and reheated in a 400°F oven for 10 to 15 minutes, or until heated through.

NUTRITIONAL INFORMATION (1 SERVING = 1 POCKET) Calories 317, Total Fat 12.9 g 20%, Saturated Fat 4.4 g 22%, Trans Fat 0.0 g, Cholesterol 16.7 mg 6%, Sodium 854.4 mg 36%, Total Carb 40.5 g 14%, Dietary Fiber 5.9 g 24%, Sugars 3 g, Added Sugars 0 g, Protein 12.7 g 25%, Vitamin D 3 mcg 1%, Calcium 331.5 mg 33%, Iron 6.1 mg 34%, Potassium 713.5 mg 20%

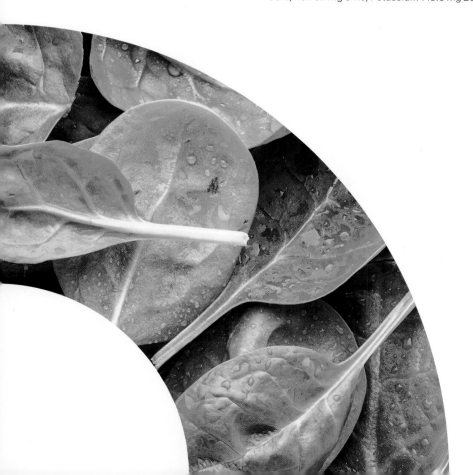

Veggie Patties with Chive Sauce

These protein-rich veggie patties, made with lentils and white beans, are as filling as any meat meal. They're a little too delicate to make on the grill, but we dare any hamburger lover to try these and not fall a little bit in love!

FOR THE PATTIES

⅓ cup black or green lentils

1 tablespoon olive oil

1 large onion, finely diced

⅔ cup finely diced zucchini

¾ teaspoon kosher salt

2 teaspoons minced garlic

½ cup drained canned white beans, mashed

2 large egg whites, lightly beaten

¼ cup dried bread crumbs

¼ cup chopped fresh parsley

¼ cup chopped scallion greens

½ teaspoon sweet paprika

¼ teaspoon red pepper flakes

FOR THE SAUCE

¾ cup plain nonfat regular yogurt (not Greek)

2 tablespoons finely minced fresh chives

1 teaspoon fresh lemon juice

½ teaspoon finely grated lemon zest

¼ teaspoon kosher salt

⅛ teaspoon freshly ground black pepper

SERVES 4   TOTAL TIME: 1 HOUR 30 MINUTES (INCLUDING CHILLING)

1. Cook the lentils: Fill a small saucepan halfway with water and bring to a boil over high heat. Lower the heat to medium, add the lentils, and cover the pan. Cook until tender but not mushy, 15 to 20 minutes. Drain well in a colander, and let cool slightly.

2. Sauté the vegetables: Heat the olive oil in a medium (9- or 10-inch) skillet over medium heat. Add the onion and zucchini and ¼ teaspoon of the salt, and cook, stirring, until lightly golden, 6 to 8 minutes.

3. Add the garlic and cook, stirring, 1 more minute.

4. Combine and chill the patty mixture: Transfer the vegetable mixture to a large bowl and add the lentils. Stir in the white beans, egg whites, bread crumbs, parsley, scallion greens, paprika, the remaining ½ teaspoon salt, and the red pepper flakes. Gently mix to combine, then press plastic wrap over the surface and chill in the refrigerator for at least 20 minutes.

5. Form and bake the patties: Preheat the oven to 425°F. Line a baking sheet with parchment and spray for 3 seconds with cooking spray. Spray your hands lightly with cooking spray.

6. Divide the lentil mixture into 8 parts, then form each part into a round patty. Space the patties out on the baking sheet with at least 1 inch between them.

7. Bake the patties until the tops are lightly crisped, 19 to 20 minutes.

continued on page 192

continued from page 191

8. Make the sauce: While the patties are baking, combine the yogurt, chives, lemon juice and zest, salt, and black pepper in a small bowl; chill until ready to use.

9. Serve the patties: Arrange the patties on a large serving platter or on 4 individual plates. Drizzle the sauce over the patties, or serve it on the side, for dipping.

NUTRITIONAL INFORMATION (1 SERVING = 2 PATTIES, PLUS 2 TABLESPOONS SAUCE) Calories 204, Total Fat 4.1 g 6%, Saturated Fat 0.6 g 3%, Trans Fat 0.0 g, Cholesterol 1.0 mg 0%, Sodium 493.3 mg 21%, Total Carb 31.8 g 11%, Dietary Fiber 5.8 g 23%, Sugars 6.3 g, Added Sugars 0 g, Protein 11.7 g 23%, Vitamin D 0.0 mcg 0%, Calcium 162.9 mg 16%, Iron 2.6 mg 14%, Potassium 454.1 mg 13%

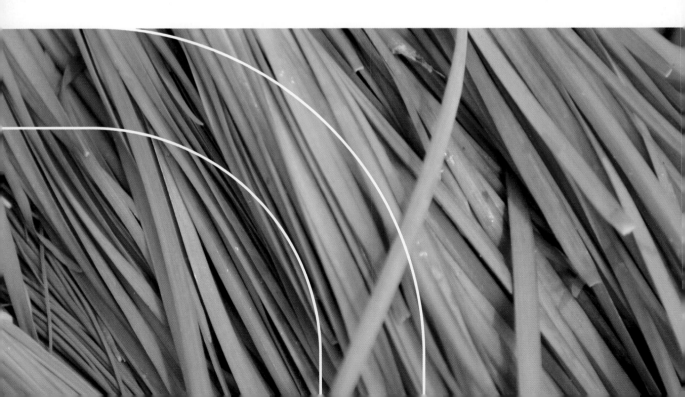

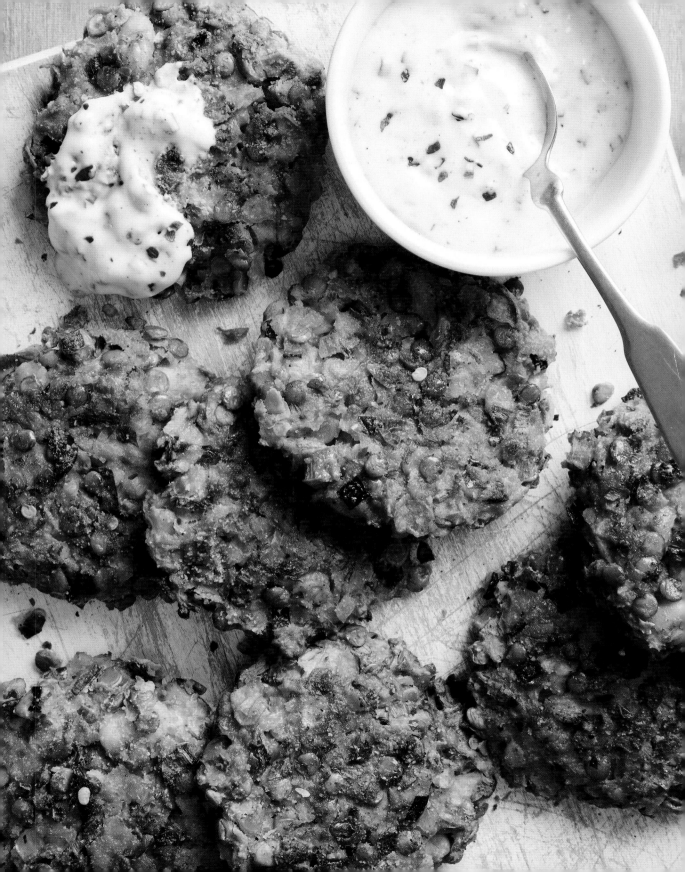

Side Dishes

Main dishes are great, but sometimes they can be a little bit short on the micronutrients—those are the vitamins, minerals, and great plant compounds that help keep us healthy. Vegetables are awesome, and you really can't eat too many of them. So, vegetable side dishes are a great way to veg-up your meals and make them more nutrient dense! In fact, we found that adding a cup of veggies to any meal both lowered the caloric density and raised the nutrient density, so we hope you'll try them all!

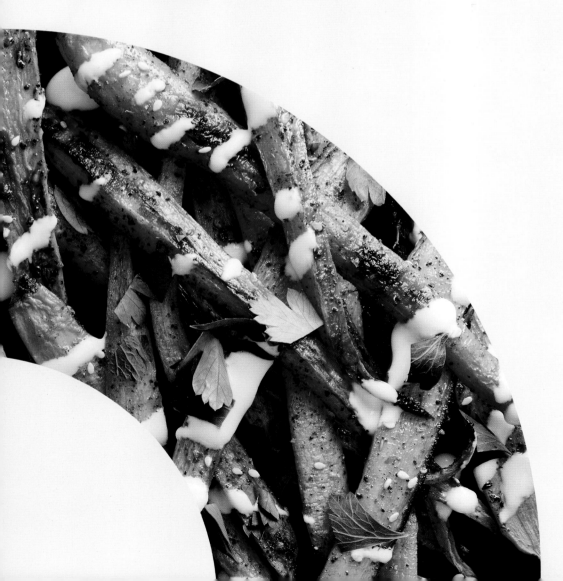

Sweet & Spicy Brussels Sprouts

These are pretty spicy if you use the full amount of gochujang, a Korean chili condiment (our recipe tester called this recipe "not for the faint at heart"). Feel free to cut the amount of gochujang in half or use a different hot sauce, if you prefer. If you *love* heat, though, this is sure to become your go-to sauce for your other favorite veggies, or for marinating meat, or for anywhere else you like to turn up the flavor.

FOR THE BRUSSELS SPROUTS

1½ pounds Brussels sprouts, ends trimmed and outer leaves removed, then halved

1 tablespoon olive oil

½ teaspoon kosher salt

¼ teaspoon freshly ground black pepper

FOR THE SAUCE

1 tablespoon honey

2 tablespoons prepared gochujang

2 teaspoons sesame seeds

1 teaspoon rice wine vinegar

SERVES 4   TOTAL TIME: 25 MINUTES

1. Roast the Brussels sprouts: Preheat the oven to 425°F. Line a rimmed baking sheet with parchment.

2. Toss the sprouts, olive oil, salt, and black pepper in a large bowl. Spread the sprouts on the baking sheet, arranging as many as possible cut side down. Roast until golden, crisp, and charred in spots, about 25 minutes, stirring halfway through cooking time.

3. Make the sauce: While the sprouts are roasting, whisk the honey, gochujang, sesame seeds, and vinegar in the bowl you used to toss the sprouts.

4. Sauce and glaze the Brussels sprouts: Carefully transfer the sprouts to the bowl with the sauce. (Keep the oven on.) Using a rubber spatula, toss to coat with the sauce, making sure all the sprouts are evenly and well coated.

5. Return the sprouts to the baking sheet, spreading again in a single layer. Roast until slightly sizzling and the sauce has been absorbed a bit, about 5 minutes.

6. Serve the sprouts: Heap the Brussels sprouts into a large serving bowl and serve hot.

NUTRITIONAL INFORMATION (1 SERVING = 1 CUP) Calories 146, Total Fat 4.7 g 7%, Saturated Fat 0.7 g 3%, Trans Fat 0.0 g, Cholesterol 0.0 mg 0%, Sodium 428.9 mg 18%, Total Carb 24 g 8%, Dietary Fiber 7.2 g 29%, Sugars 11.2 g, Added Sugars 0 g, Protein 6 g 12%, Vitamin D 0.0 mcg 0%, Calcium 93.2 mg 9%, Iron 2.5 mg 14%, Potassium 671.4 mg 19%

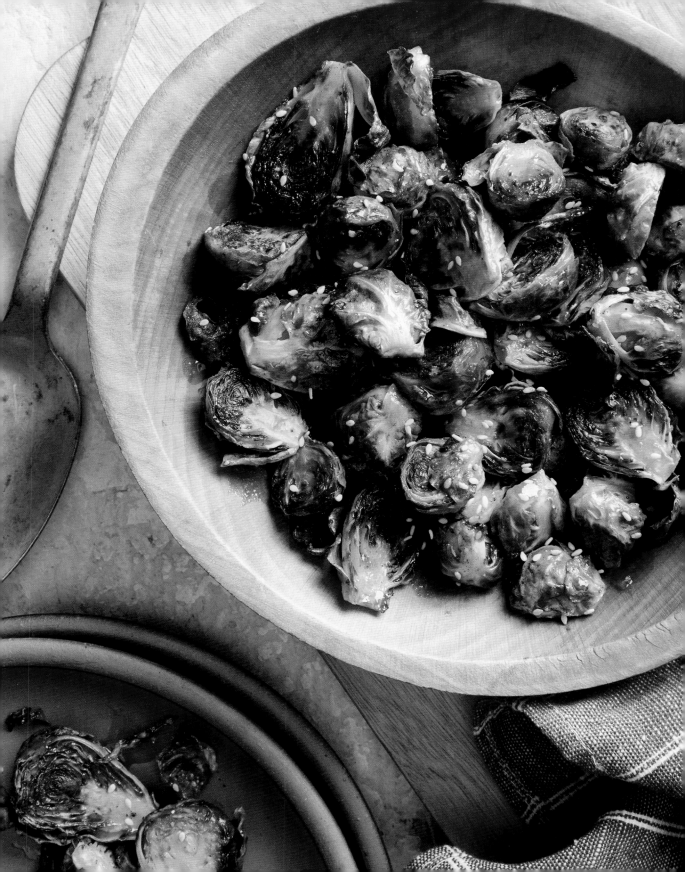

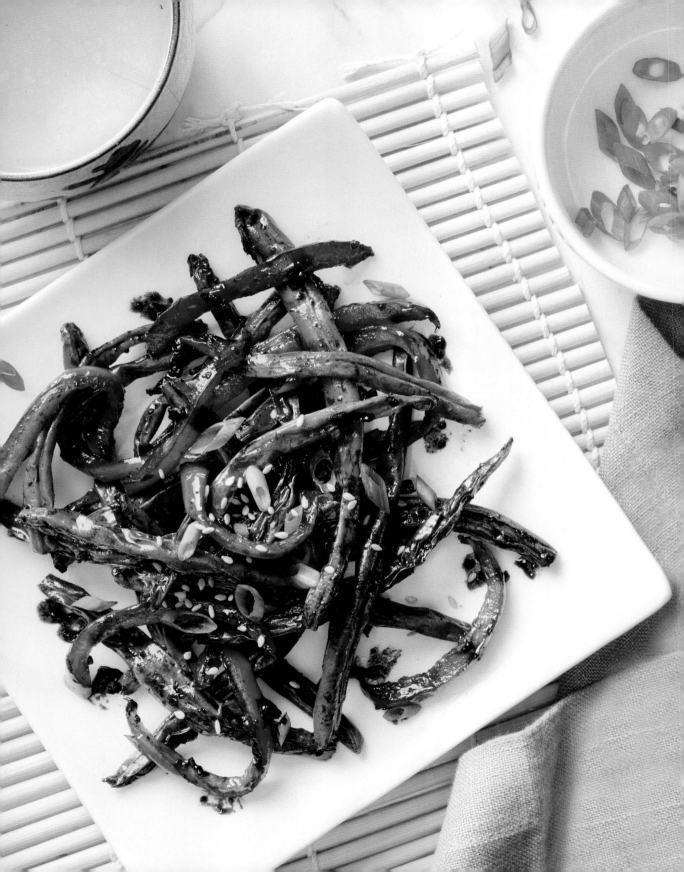

Green Beans & Red Pepper in Black Bean Sauce

A tip for making simple recipes taste really special is to include spices, sauces, and condiments with exotic flavors. One of our faves is black bean sauce, a paste made of fermented black beans that lends a sweet, salty, savory, surprising flavor that will have your family saying, "Ooh, what's in this? Can I have some more?" Isn't that what we all want to hear when we put dinner on the table?

FOR THE VEGETABLES

1 pound fresh green beans, trimmed

4 teaspoons olive oil

½ teaspoon kosher salt

1 red bell pepper, cored, seeded, and thinly sliced

FOR THE SAUCE

2½ tablespoons Chinese black bean sauce

2 tablespoons finely minced fresh ginger

1½ tablespoons rice vinegar

1 tablespoon reduced-sodium soy sauce

3 garlic cloves, minced

2 teaspoons toasted sesame oil

2 teaspoons pure maple syrup

FOR SERVING

3 tablespoons sliced scallion greens

1 teaspoon toasted sesame seeds

SERVES 4 TOTAL TIME: 25 MINUTES

1. Roast the green beans and red pepper: Preheat the oven to 500°F.

2. Arrange the beans on a rimmed baking sheet. Drizzle with 2 teaspoons of the olive oil, sprinkle with ¼ teaspoon of the salt, and toss to coat. Roast the beans for 10 minutes.

3. Remove the baking sheet from the oven, stir, and move the beans to one side. Add the red pepper and drizzle with the remaining 2 teaspoons olive oil and ¼ teaspoon salt. Toss to coat.

4. Return the baking sheet to the oven and continue to roast until the beans are browned and shriveled and the red pepper is soft, about another 10 minutes.

5. Make the sauce and add to the vegetables: While the beans and peppers are roasting, whisk together the black bean sauce, ginger, vinegar, soy sauce, garlic, sesame oil, and maple syrup in a small bowl.

6. Remove the vegetables from the oven, reduce the heat to 450°F, and pour the sauce over the beans and pepper. Toss lightly, then return to the oven and roast until the beans absorb a bit of the sauce, 1 to 2 minutes.

7. Serve the vegetables: Transfer the vegetables to a large serving platter, and garnish with the scallions and sesame seeds. Serve family style.

NUTRITIONAL INFORMATION (1 SERVING = GENEROUS ¾ CUP) Calories 153, Total Fat 7.7 g 12%, Saturated Fat 1.1 g 6%, Trans Fat 0.0 g, Cholesterol 0.0 mg 0%, Sodium 769.1 mg 32%, Total Carb 19.3 g 6%, Dietary Fiber 4 g 16%, Sugars 11.3 g, Added Sugars 0 g, Protein 3.7 g 7%, Vitamin D 0.0 mcg 0%, Calcium 55.7 mg 6%, Iron 1.7 mg 10%, Potassium 345.6 mg 10%

Mushroom-Stuffed Lettuce Cups

Larb is a traditional salad popular in Thailand and Laos, made with chopped seasoned meat and herbs and served with papaya salad and sticky rice. We've significantly lightened it up and made it plant-based by replacing the meat with mushrooms and by serving the larb in lettuce cups. (If you want to make this totally plant based, use vegan Worcestershire instead of regular Worcestershire or fish sauce.) This makes a fancy vegetarian side dish, or even a light lunch. Wear kitchen gloves when you chop the Thai chilies if you decide to use them—they are hot!

1 head butter lettuce (such as Boston bibb) or other soft head lettuce

1 pound fresh button mushrooms, stems removed

¼ cup sliced scallion greens

¼ cup finely minced red onion

¼ cup chopped fresh cilantro

¼ cup chopped fresh mint

¼ cup chopped Thai basil or Italian basil

Grated zest and juice of 1 lime (1 teaspoon zest and ¼ cup juice)

1 tablespoon Thai fish sauce or low-sodium Worcestershire sauce

1 teaspoon light brown sugar or palm sugar

¼ teaspoon red pepper flakes or thinly sliced Thai (bird's-eye) chili, or more for serving (optional)

SERVES 4 TOTAL TIME: 15 MINUTES

1. Make the cups: Use a small knife to cut into the core of the lettuce. Gently separate the leaves and choose 12 small, cup-shaped leaves.

2. Make the filling: Working in 2 batches, pulse the mushrooms in a food processor until very finely chopped, 20 to 25 pulses (don't process for too long, or they will turn to liquid). Transfer the mushrooms to a large bowl and add the scallion greens, red onion, cilantro, mint, and basil.

3. In a small bowl, whisk the lime juice and zest, fish sauce, brown sugar, and ¼ teaspoon red pepper flakes, if using. Add to the mushroom mixture and gently toss.

4. Assemble the cups and serve: Divide the filling among the 12 lettuce cups. Nestle 3 cups together on each of 4 plates. Garnish with additional red pepper flakes and serve.

NUTRITIONAL INFORMATION (1 SERVING = 3 LETTUCE CUPS, WITH ¼ CUP FILLING IN EACH) Calories 46, Total Fat 0.6 g 1%, Saturated Fat 0.1 g 0%, Trans Fat 0.0 g, Cholesterol 0.0 mg 0%, Sodium 364.1 mg 15%, Total Carb 8.5 g 3%, Dietary Fiber 2 g 8%, Sugars 4.6 g, Added Sugars 0 g, Protein 4.7 g 9%, Vitamin D 8 mcg 2%, Calcium 31.6 mg 3%, Iron 1.3 mg 7%, Potassium 518.5 mg 15%

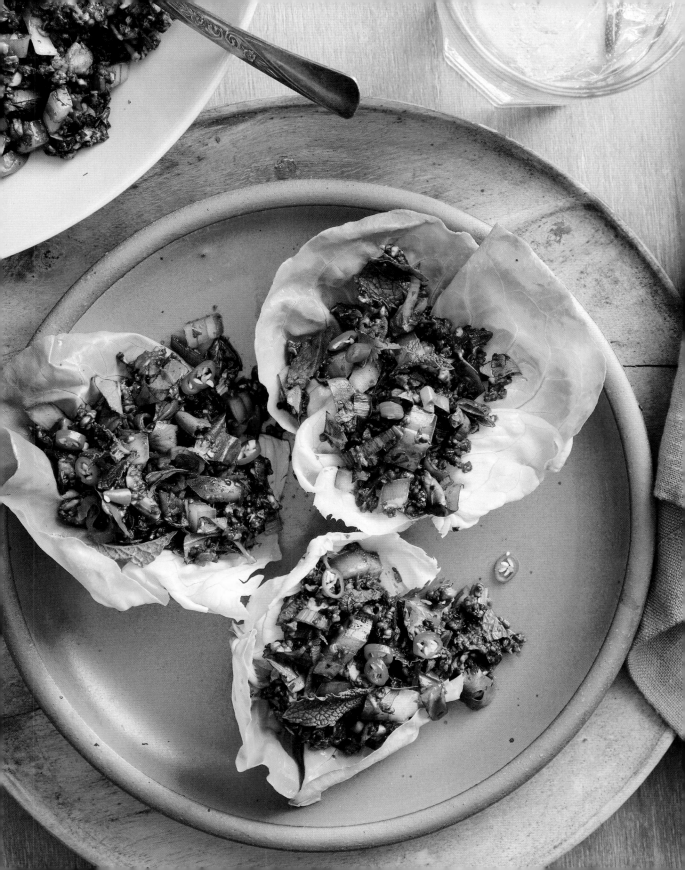

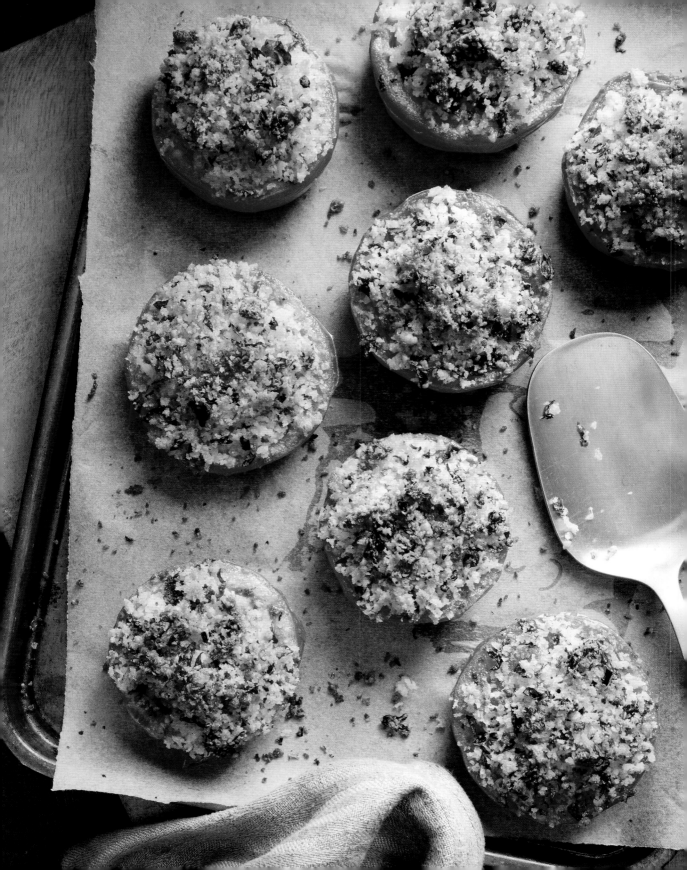

Roasted Tomato Cups with Bread Crumbs

This is ultimate comfort food, spiked with high-flavor ingredients like Parmesan cheese and anchovies (seriously, give those little fishes a chance to impress you with their flavor; you won't be mad about the boost of nutrients they offer!), so you can enjoy a little of this and feel supremely satisfied.

½ cup panko or other bread crumbs

¼ cup very finely grated Parmigiano-Reggiano cheese

2 tablespoons chopped fresh parsley, plus more for garnish

1 or 2 oil-packed anchovies, drained (but not patted dry), very finely chopped

1 tablespoon olive oil (or oil from anchovy can, for extra flavor)

1 teaspoon finely grated lemon zest

¼ teaspoon red pepper flakes

¼ teaspoon salt

⅛ teaspoon freshly ground black pepper

6 vine-ripened medium tomatoes (1¼ pounds), cored and halved crosswise

SERVES 6 TOTAL TIME: 20 MINUTES

1. Preheat the oven to 425°F. Line a rimmed baking sheet with parchment.

2. Prepare the crumbs: Combine the panko, cheese, parsley, anchovies, olive oil, lemon zest, red pepper flakes, salt, and pepper in a medium bowl and toss until the ingredients are well combined.

3. Bake the tomatoes: Arrange the tomato halves, cut side up, on the baking sheet and divide the topping among them (1 heaping tablespoon per half). Roast until the tomatoes soften slightly and the crumbs are golden and crisp, 12 to 15 minutes.

4. Serve the tomatoes: Transfer the tomato halves to a large serving platter or to 6 individual plates and serve hot or at room temperature.

NUTRITIONAL INFORMATION (1 SERVING = 2 TOMATO HALVES) Calories 66, Total Fat 3.9 g 6%, Saturated Fat 1.4 g 7%, Trans Fat 0.0 g, Cholesterol 4.7 mg 2%, Sodium 161.1 mg 7%, Total Carb 5.5 g 2%, Dietary Fiber 1.3 g 5%, Sugars 2.6 g, Added Sugars 0 g, Protein 2.9 g 6%, Vitamin D 0.5 mcg 0%, Calcium 63.5 mg 6%, Iron 0.5 mg 2%, Potassium 235.9 mg 7%

Scallion-y Cauliflower & Brown Rice

6 cups fresh cauliflower florets (1¼ to 1½ pounds)

2 tablespoons olive oil

4 scallions, thinly sliced, white and green parts kept separate

1 tablespoon minced garlic

¾ teaspoon kosher salt, plus more for seasoning

1 cup cooked brown rice

2 teaspoons toasted sesame oil

Toasted slivered almonds and/or lemon zest, for garnish

Here's a great way to use up leftover brown rice—makes it feel like it's a whole new dish. This recipe is a quick and easy side dish that pairs well with a protein like fish or chicken, but you could also add toss in more veggies and enjoy it for a fast lunch or dinner! It's got the savory flavor and satisfying texture of brown rice, with the lightness of what has been termed cauliflower rice. It's the best of both worlds.

SERVES 4   TOTAL TIME: 30 MINUTES

1. Make the cauliflower rice: Grate the cauliflower florets on the large holes of a box grater or pulse in a food processor in batches until the cauliflower resembles rice.

2. Sauté the cauliflower rice: Heat 1 tablespoon of the olive oil in a large (12-inch) nonstick skillet over medium heat. Add the scallion whites and garlic and cook, stirring, until fragrant, about 2 minutes. Add the remaining tablespoon olive oil to the skillet, then add the cauliflower rice and ¾ teaspoon of the salt. Cook, stirring, until the cauliflower softens and loses most of its moisture, 6 to 7 minutes.

3. Add the brown rice and serve: Add the brown rice to the skillet, followed by the sesame oil, and cook, stirring, until everything is combined and looks unified, about 2 minutes. Stir in the scallion greens, cook 1 more minute, and season to taste with more salt.

4. Divide the stir-fry among 4 bowls or plates and serve hot, garnished with the almonds and lemon zest, if desired.

NUTRITIONAL INFORMATION (1 SERVING = 1 CUP) Calories 183, Total Fat 9.9 g 15%, Saturated Fat 1.4 g 7%, Trans Fat 0.0 g, Cholesterol 0.0 mg 0%, Sodium 329.1 mg 14%, Total Carb 21.3 g 7%, Dietary Fiber 4.5 g 18%, Sugars 3.5 g, Added Sugars 0 g, Protein 4.6 g 9%, Vitamin D 0.0 mcg 0%, Calcium 55.1 mg 6%, Iron 1.2 mg 7%, Potassium 568.9 mg 16%

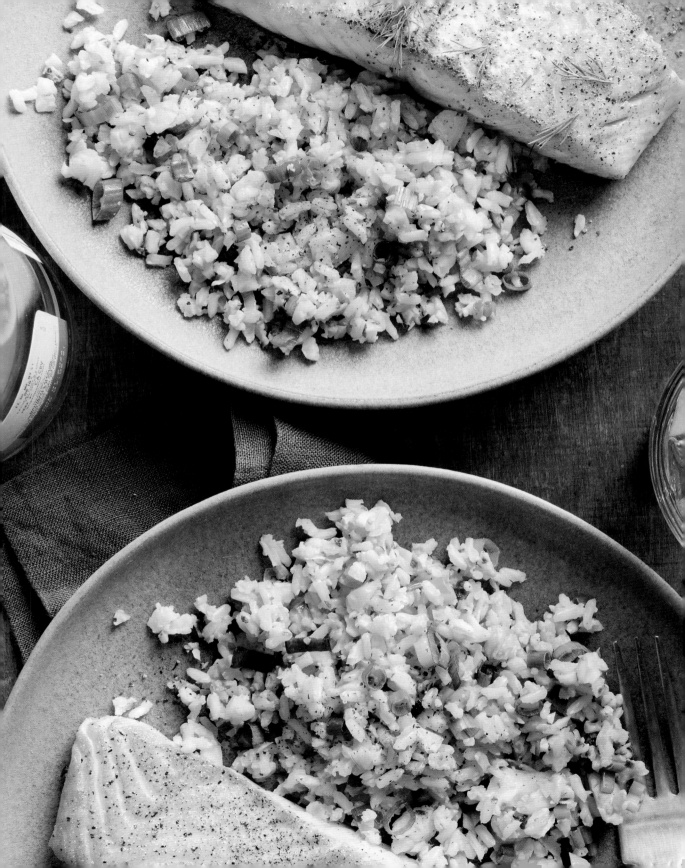

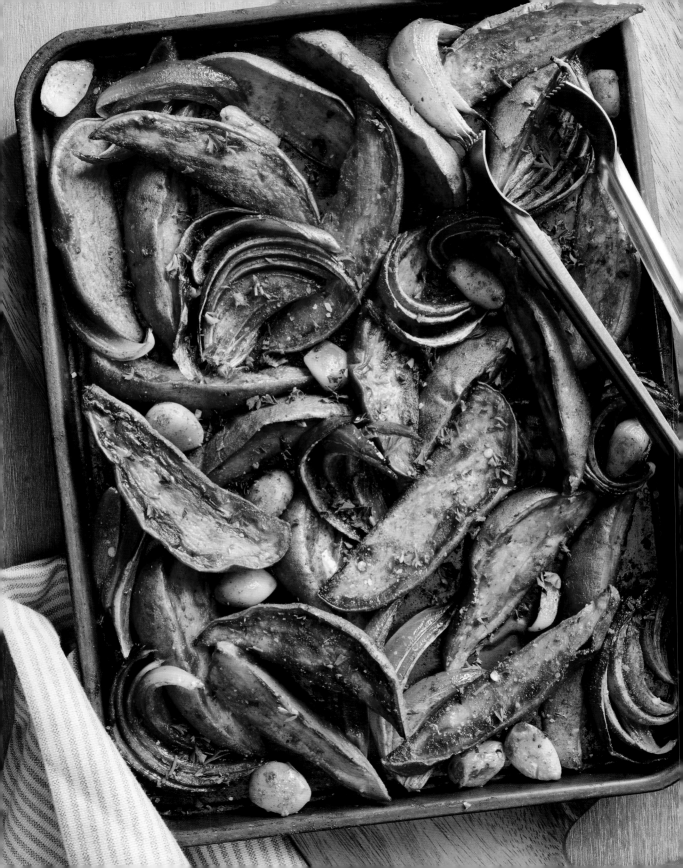

Spicy Sweet Potato Fries

Roasting brings out the luxurious sweetness of both sweet potatoes and onions, which is further enhanced with sweet spices and a bit of zing. These are no ordinary sweet potato fries. They are superior in taste, nutritional value, and caloric density—note that this is a green food!

2 tablespoons olive oil

1 teaspoon sweet paprika

1 teaspoon ground cumin

1 teaspoon ground coriander

1 teaspoon kosher salt, plus more for seasoning

½ teaspoon cayenne (or red pepper flakes), plus more for seasoning

1½ pounds sweet potatoes, scrubbed and cut into ½-inch-thick wedges or slices

1 large red onion, cut into ¼-inch-thick wedges

15 large garlic cloves

2 tablespoons water

2 tablespoons chopped fresh parsley

SERVES 6   TOTAL TIME: 1 HOUR

1. Arrange a rack in the top third of the oven. Preheat the oven to 425°F.

2. Flavor the sweet potato wedges: Whisk the olive oil, paprika, cumin, coriander, salt, and cayenne in a large bowl. Add the sweet potatoes, onion, and garlic, and toss to coat.

3. Transfer the potato mixture to a rimmed baking sheet. Add the water and seal tightly with foil.

4. Roast the vegetables: Roast the vegetables for 20 minutes, then remove the foil and continue to roast until the sweet potatoes are soft in the center and crisped on the outside, and the onion and garlic are softened and golden, another 25 to 30 minutes.

5. If you like your vegetables more charred, turn on the broiler and broil until the potatoes, onion, and garlic char and crisp, watching to make sure they don't burn, 3 to 4 minutes.

6. Serve the fries: Transfer the fries to a large serving bowl, season with more salt and cayenne, if desired, and garnish with the parsley. Serve at once.

NUTRITIONAL INFORMATION (1 SERVING = SCANT 1 CUP) Calories 103, Total Fat 5 g 8%, Saturated Fat 0.8 g 4%, Trans Fat 0.0 g, Cholesterol 0.0 mg 0%, Sodium 260.6 mg 11%, Total Carb 12.5 g 4%, Dietary Fiber 3.1 g 12%, Sugars 1.2 g, Added Sugars 0 g, Protein 5.5 g 11%, Vitamin D 0.0 mcg 0%, Calcium 60.7 mg 6%, Iron 1.5 mg 8%, Potassium 640.1 mg 18%

Sweet & Spicy Sautéed Spinach

Of all the dark leafy greens available to us in the market, spinach is a favorite because it has a mild taste compared to other, more bitter greens—and it's good both raw and cooked. The combination of sweetness from the golden raisins here and the spiciness from the jalapeño makes this dish both unusual and addictive. Just remember to wear gloves while you're chopping those jalapeños, and don't touch your eyes or nose! If you want to tone down the spiciness, cut away all the white parts (pith) from the jalapeños and take out all the seeds. The pith and seeds are the spiciest parts.

2 tablespoons pine nuts

1 tablespoon olive oil

2 tablespoons finely chopped red bell pepper

5 garlic cloves, thinly sliced

1 jalapeño, thinly sliced (seeded, if desired)

2 tablespoons golden raisins

1 pound baby spinach

½ teaspoon kosher salt

1 small lemon

SERVES 4 TOTAL TIME: 15 MINUTES

1. Toast the pine nuts: Heat a large (12-inch) skillet over medium heat. Add the pine nuts and cook, stirring every minute or so, until golden in spots and fragrant, 5 to 6 minutes. Transfer to a plate to cool.

2. Sauté the vegetables: Add the olive oil to the skillet, then add the bell pepper, garlic, and jalapeño and cook, stirring, until lightly golden and fragrant, about 1 minute. Add the raisins to the skillet, then raise the heat to medium-high.

3. Working in 3 batches, add the spinach and cook, stirring, until the spinach is wilted but not completely limp, 3 to 4 minutes total. (Tongs are a handy tool to grab the wilted spinach from the bottom of the pan and place on top of the pile so it doesn't get overcooked.) Stir in the salt.

4. Serve the spinach: Using tongs or a slotted spoon, transfer the spinach to a large platter, then zest the lemon directly over the spinach. Halve the lemon and squeeze the juice over the spinach as well, as desired (1 to 2 tablespoons juice). Sprinkle with the pine nuts.

5. Divide the spinach among 4 serving bowls and serve warm or at room temperature.

NUTRITIONAL INFORMATION (1 SERVING = ABOUT ¾ CUP) Calories 113, Total Fat 6.9 g 11%, Saturated Fat 0.8 g 4%, Trans Fat 0.0 g, Cholesterol 0.0 mg 0%, Sodium 276.5 mg 12%, Total Carb 11.8 g 4%, Dietary Fiber 3.3 g 13%, Sugars 4.5 g, Added Sugars 0 g, Protein 4.4 g 9%, Vitamin D 0.0 mcg 0%, Calcium 126.2 mg 13%, Iron 3.5 mg 20%, Potassium 748.6 mg 21%

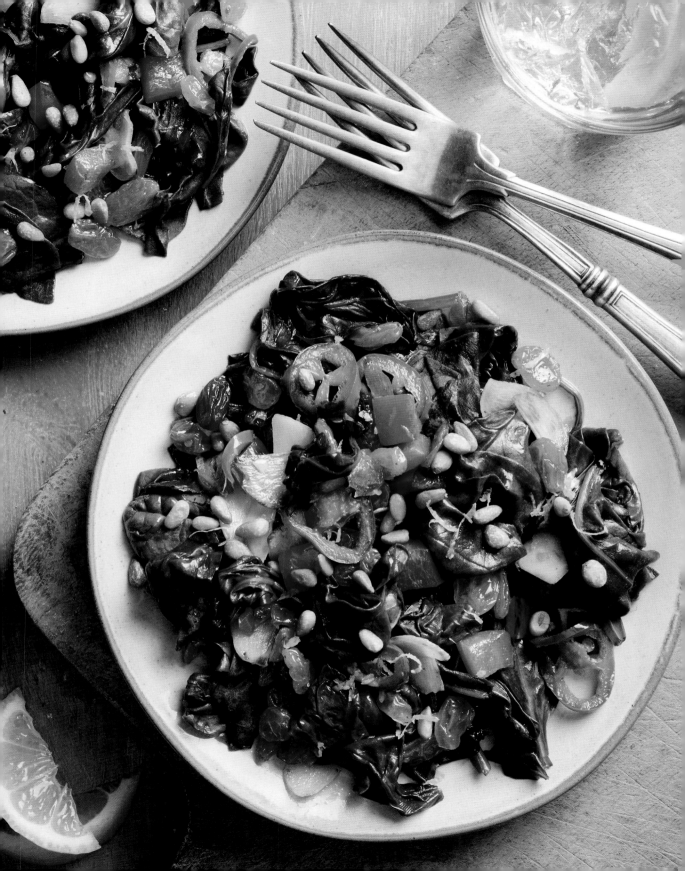

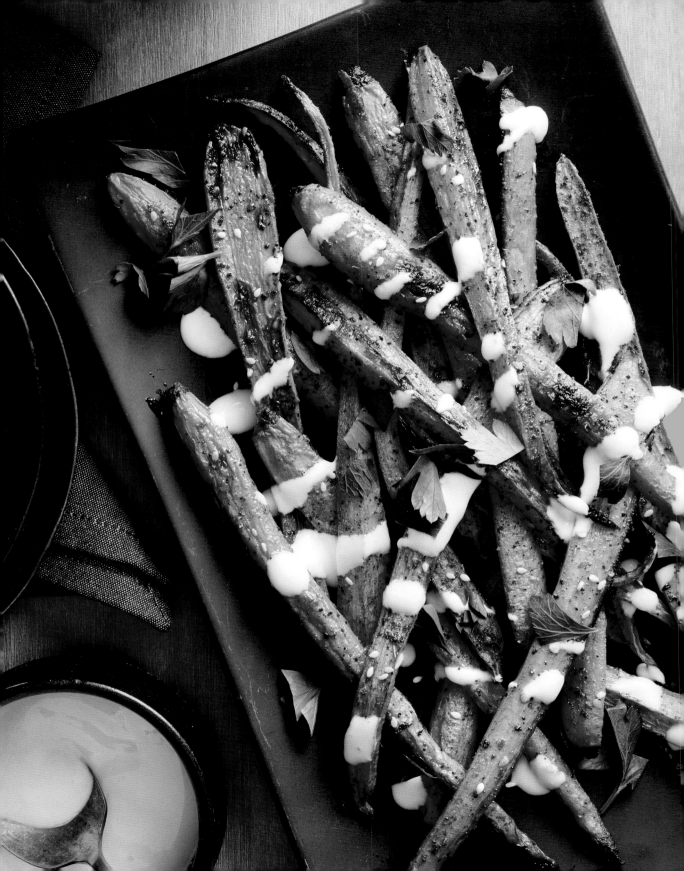

Za'atar Roasted Carrots with Lemony Yogurt

Za'atar is a Middle Eastern herb and spice mixture that contains herbs like dried oregano and thyme, spices like cumin, coriander, and sumac, plus sesame seeds. You can find it in the spice aisle of some groceries or online; trust us—you want to get to know this delicious, tangy mixture. Preserved lemons—basically, pickled lemons—are a tart and salty condiment often used in North African and South Asian dishes. If you can't find preserved lemon, you can substitute fresh lemon, and it will still taste delicious.

2 pounds thin carrots (ideally no more than 1 inch in diameter at the top), trimmed

1½ tablespoons olive oil

2½ tablespoons za'atar

½ teaspoon kosher salt

½ teaspoon freshly ground black pepper

½ cup plain nonfat regular yogurt (not Greek)

1 tablespoon finely chopped preserved lemon

2 tablespoons chopped fresh parsley

SERVES 4 TOTAL TIME: 45 MINUTES

1. Roast the carrots: Preheat the oven to 425°F.

2. Halve the carrots lengthwise, then halve the thicker parts again. Spread the carrots on a rimmed baking sheet. Drizzle with the olive oil, then sprinkle with the za'atar, salt, and pepper, and toss to coat.

3. Roast the carrots, tossing every 10 minutes, until charred and shriveled, 30 to 35 minutes total.

4. Make the sauce: While the carrots are roasting, stir together the yogurt and preserved lemon in a small bowl.

5. Serve the carrots: Transfer the roasted carrots to a large serving platter and drizzle the yogurt over.

6. Garnish with the parsley and serve hot or at room temperature.

NUTRITIONAL INFORMATION (1 SERVING = 7 TO 8 PIECES) Calories 164, Total Fat 6.1 g 9%, Saturated Fat 0.9 g 4%, Trans Fat 0.0 g, Cholesterol 1.4 mg 0%, Sodium 585.4 mg 24%, Total Carb 23.8 g 8%, Dietary Fiber 6.5 g 26%, Sugars 12.4 g, Added Sugars 0 g, Protein 5.1 g 10%, Vitamin D 0.0 mcg 0%, Calcium 110 mg 11%, Iron 0.9 mg 5%, Potassium 780.2 mg 22%

Onion & Sweet Potato Gratin

If you want to get fancy and old-school at the same time (#classic), try this silky, tender, cheesy gratin made with sweet potatoes and white onions. This is a great dish for serving during the holidays, or any time you're in the mood for a little comfort food.

FOR THE ONIONS

2 pounds medium sweet onions, halved and cut into ¼-inch half-moons

1 teaspoon kosher salt

6 fresh thyme sprigs

1½ tablespoons olive oil

FOR THE SAUCE

2½ cups 1 percent milk

4 tablespoons white whole wheat or rice flour

½ teaspoon salt

½ cup finely shredded Parmigiano-Reggiano cheese

1 tablespoon unsalted butter

2 teaspoons snipped fresh sage (or 1 teaspoon dried)

⅛ teaspoon grated nutmeg

FOR THE GRATIN

1 pound sweet potatoes, peeled and thinly sliced

SERVES 9 TOTAL TIME: 2 HOURS 50 MINUTES

1. Preheat the oven to 400°F. Spray a rimmed baking sheet with cooking spray.

2. Prepare the onions: Arrange the onion slices on the baking dish and sprinkle with ½ teaspoon of the salt. Add the thyme sprigs, seal tightly with foil, and steam-roast until the onions have softened and can be pierced with a fork but are still firm, about 20 minutes. Pour off any accumulated liquid. Adjust the oven to 350°F.

3. Brush the tops of the onions with the oil, season with the remaining ½ teaspoon salt, and roast uncovered until the onions are very soft and lightly golden, about 20 minutes. Discard the thyme and pour off any accumulated liquid.

4. Make the sauce: In a small saucepan off the heat, whisk together the milk, flour, and salt for 2 minutes, until the mixture is smooth. Turn the heat on to medium-high and bring the milk mixture to a boil, then reduce the heat to medium-low and simmer until the mixture thickens, 2 to 3 minutes, whisking constantly.

5. Remove the saucepan from the heat and stir in ¼ cup of the cheese, the butter, sage, and nutmeg.

6. Assemble and bake the gratin: Preheat the oven to 350°F. Spray a 9-inch square baking dish with cooking spray.

continued on page 214

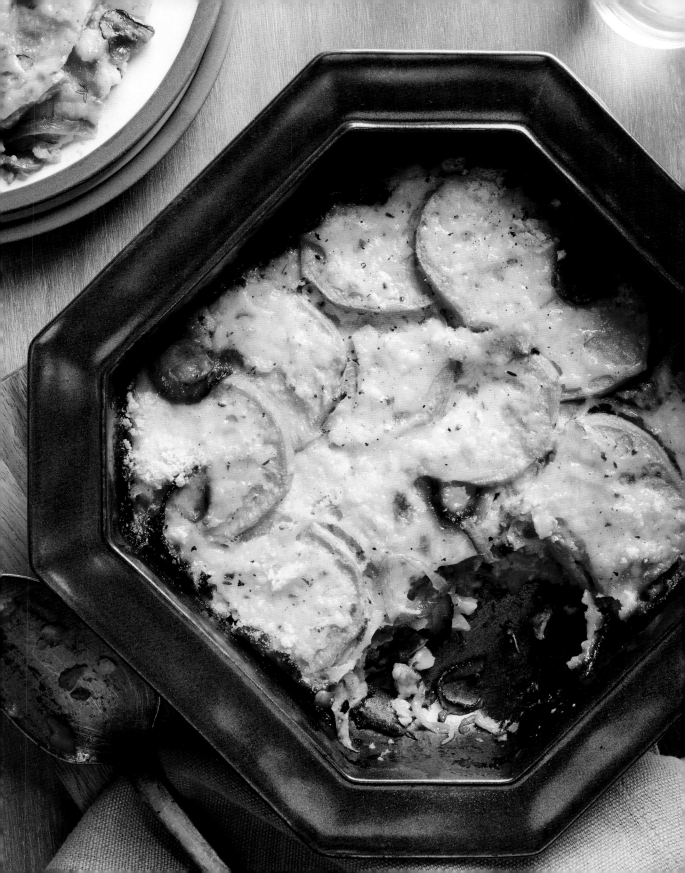

continued from page 212

7. Spoon ½ cup of the sauce onto the bottom of the dish. Arrange half the onions in a layer, then drizzle ½ cup sauce over the onions. Add another layer of the sweet potatoes, overlapping them slightly in a shingle pattern. Drizzle ½ cup of the sauce over the sweet potatoes, then sprinkle with 2 tablespoons of the cheese. Repeat one more time with the onions, sweet potatoes, sauce, and the remaining 2 tablespoons cheese.

8. Cover tightly with foil, and bake the gratin until the potatoes are soft, about 45 minutes.

9. Serve the gratin: Allow the gratin to cool slightly, then cut into 9 pieces, each about 3 inches square. Transfer the squares to 9 individual plates and serve while still warm.

NUTRITIONAL INFORMATION (1 SERVING = 3-INCH SQUARE) Calories 182, Total Fat 6.2 g 10%, Saturated Fat 3 g 15%, Trans Fat 0.1 g, Cholesterol 11.7 mg 4%, Sodium 271.3 mg 11%, Total Carb 25.8 g 9%, Dietary Fiber 3.2 g 13%, Sugars 6.5 g, Added Sugars 0 g, Protein 6.9 g 14%, Vitamin D 1.0 mcg 0%, Calcium 176 mg 18%, Iron 1.0 mg 5%, Potassium 285.6 mg 8%

CHEF'S TIP *What's a mandoline? It's a handy tool for making perfectly even slices of potato.*

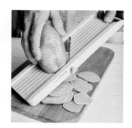

Asparagus with Roasted Red Pepper Sauce & Grated Egg

This pretty dish uses grated egg—yes, that's a thing—over crisp green asparagus and a bright red pepper sauce (#colorstory). If you've never seen this technique before, get ready for your new favorite way to eat eggs! This would be a festive dish during the holidays, but it's probably best in spring, when asparagus is at its seasonal peak. Either way, this side dish is as delicious as it is decorative.

FOR THE EGGS AND
VEGETABLES

4 large eggs

2 teaspoons kosher salt

2 large red bell peppers, cored, seeded, and halved

1 large bunch asparagus (about 1 pound), tough ends trimmed

2 garlic cloves

1 tablespoon olive oil

¼ teaspoon kosher salt

1 2-ounce jar water-packed capers, drained, rinsed, and patted dry

FOR THE ROASTED
RED PEPPER SAUCE

2 teaspoons olive oil

½ teaspoon kosher salt, plus more as needed

½ teaspoon fresh lemon juice

¼ teaspoon red pepper flakes

SERVES 4   TOTAL TIME: 90 MINUTES (INCLUDING COOLING)

1. Prepare the eggs: Fill a medium bowl with 2 cups of ice cubes and add 2 cups of cold water.

2. Place the eggs in a small saucepan, cover with 2 inches of water, season with the salt, bring to a boil over medium-high heat, then reduce the heat to medium-low and simmer until the eggs are cooked through, about 9 minutes.

3. Use a slotted spoon to transfer the eggs to the ice water, deliberately cracking them slightly so some water permeates the shells. Chill for 5 minutes, then peel under cold running water.

4. Roast the vegetables: Preheat the oven to 450°F.

5. Line a rimmed baking sheet with parchment and arrange the pepper halves. Roast until puffed and blackened in spots, 35 to 40 minutes total.

6. While the peppers are roasting, arrange the asparagus, garlic cloves, and capers on another rimmed baking sheet. Drizzle with the olive oil, sprinkle with the salt, and shake to coat lightly.

continued on page 217

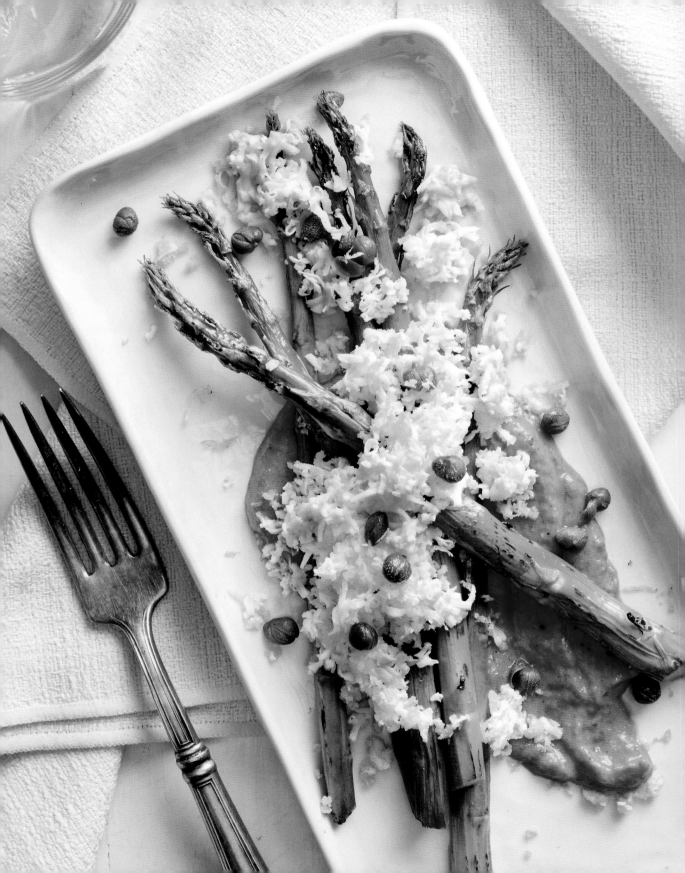

continued from page 215

7. During the last 15 minutes of roasting the peppers, add the asparagus baking sheet to the oven and roast until wilted and charred and the capers are crisp, 14 to 15 minutes.

8. When all the vegetables are done roasting, use tongs to place the peppers in a bowl, cover tightly with plastic wrap, and let cool for 30 minutes.

9. Peel the peppers and make the sauce: Uncover the peppers. Working over the sink, remove and discard blackened peels. Place the peppers in a bullet-style blender or small bowl of a food processor, and add the olive oil, the roasted garlic cloves, the salt, lemon juice, and red pepper flakes. Blend until smooth and creamy, 15 to 20 seconds.

10. Serve the dish: Spoon ¼ cup of the sauce onto each of 4 individual plates. Divide the asparagus among the plates. Using a microplane grater, finely grate one egg over each plate, and top each with 2 teaspoons of the crispy capers. Serve at room temperature.

NUTRITIONAL INFORMATION (1 SERVING = 1 CUP) Calories 174, Total Fat 13.2 g 20%, Saturated Fat 2.7 g 14%, Trans Fat 0.1 g, Cholesterol 186 mg 62%, Sodium 699.6 mg 29%, Total Carb 6.3 g 2%, Dietary Fiber 2 g 8%, Sugars 3.7 g, Added Sugars 0 g, Protein 7.4 g 15%, Vitamin D 41 mcg 10%, Calcium 40 mg 4%, Iron 1.4 mg 8%, Potassium 252.2 mg 7%

CHEF'S TIP *Use a microplane or box grater to grate the hard-boiled eggs over the salad.*

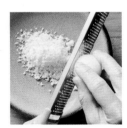

Glazed Squash with Hazelnuts

This hearty winter salad contains filling butternut squash glazed with sweet pomegranate molasses, a popular flavoring in Middle Eastern cuisine. If you can't find it in your local market, look online—once you try this tasty sweetener, we predict you'll want to use it on everything!

FOR THE SQUASH

¼ cup hazelnuts

4 cups (1¼ pounds) cubed butternut squash

1 tablespoon olive oil

½ teaspoon kosher salt

½ teaspoon ground cumin

¼ teaspoon freshly ground black pepper

1 tablespoon pomegranate molasses

FOR THE DRESSING

2 tablespoons olive oil

2 tablespoons water

1 tablespoon pomegranate molasses

1 teaspoon finely minced shallot

1 teaspoon Dijon mustard

¼ teaspoon kosher salt

¼ teaspoon black pepper

FOR THE SALAD

5 cups baby arugula leaves

½ cup thinly sliced red onion

¼ cup pomegranate seeds (arils)

Kosher salt and freshly ground black pepper

SERVES 4   TOTAL TIME: 40 MINUTES

1. Toast the hazelnuts and bake the squash: Preheat the oven to 400°F. Adjust the racks to have one in the upper third and one in the lower third of the oven.

2. Arrange the hazelnuts on a rimmed baking sheet.

3. In a large bowl, toss the squash with the olive oil, salt, cumin, and pepper, and transfer to a large roasting pan.

4. Place both the baking sheet and the roasting pan in the oven and roast until the hazelnuts are golden, 7 to 8 minutes.

5. Remove the hazelnuts from the oven, but continue to roast the squash until softened with some charred edges, another 15 minutes (23 to 25 minutes total). Chop the hazelnuts.

6. Remove the squash from the oven (leave oven turned on), drizzle with the pomegranate molasses, stir gently to coat, then return to the oven. Roast until slightly caramelized, about 5 more minutes.

7. Make the dressing: While the squash is roasting, combine the olive oil, water, pomegranate molasses, shallot, mustard, salt, and pepper in a small jar. Seal with the lid and shake until creamy, about 10 seconds.

8. Assemble and serve the salad: Arrange the arugula on a large platter and top with the roasted squash, chopped hazelnuts, red onion, and pomegranate seeds. Drizzle with the dressing. Season to taste with salt and pepper. Serve family style.

NUTRITIONAL INFORMATION (1 SERVING = 3 CUPS SQUASH, PLUS GREENS) Calories 258, Total Fat 14.9 g 23%, Saturated Fat 1.8 g 9%, Trans Fat 0.0 g, Cholesterol 0.0 mg 0%, Sodium 320.7 mg 13%, Total Carb 31 g 10%, Dietary Fiber 4.7 g 19%, Sugars 12.8 g, Added Sugars 0 g, Protein 4.6 g 9%, Vitamin D 0.0 mcg 0%, Calcium 113.7 mg 11%, Iron 1.8 mg 10%, Potassium 656.4 mg 19%

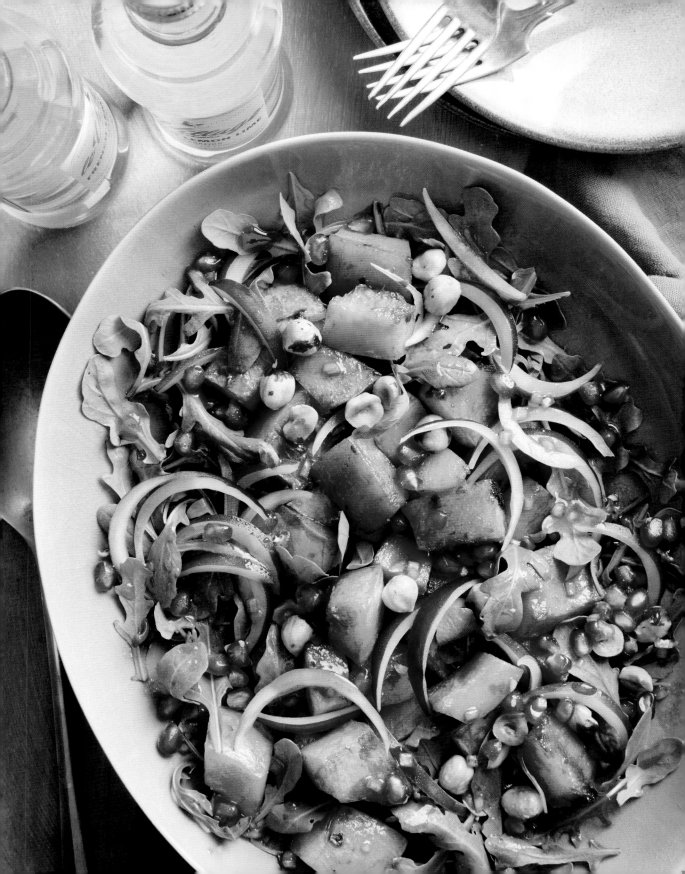

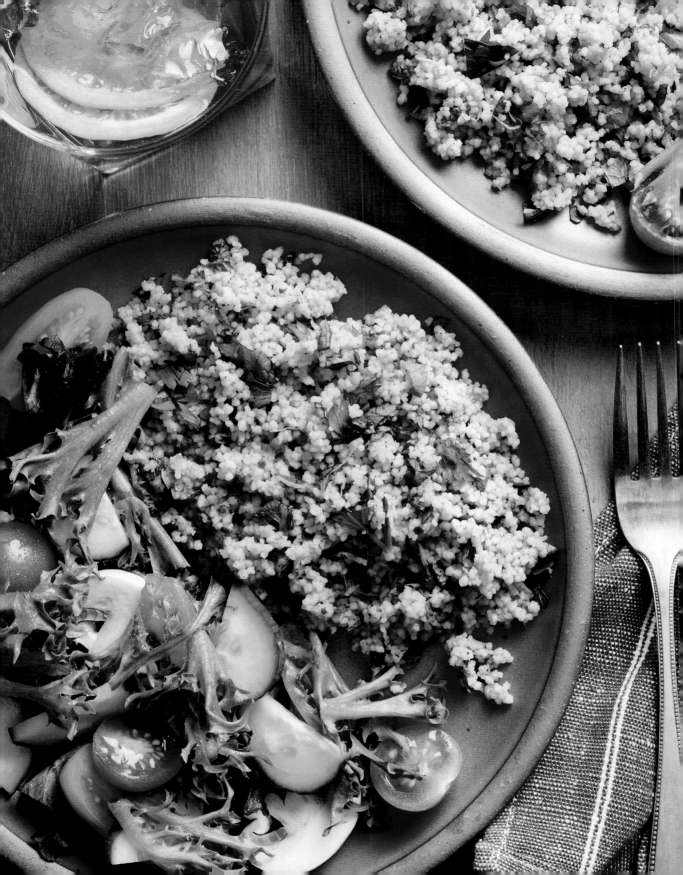

Herbed Whole-Grain Couscous

Couscous looks like a grain, but it's actually a pasta. It cooks in a jif, and with a sprinkling of herbs, it just might be one of the easiest side dishes in our arsenal. It also goes with just about anything: meat, poultry, fish, tofu—you can even use it to top your salad. This recipe is also 100 percent plant-based and 100 percent delish.

1¼ cups low-sodium vegetable broth

¾ cup whole-grain couscous

1 tablespoon olive oil

1 tablespoon fresh lemon juice

1 teaspoon finely grated lemon zest

¼ cup chopped fresh herbs of choice (basil, parsley, dill, cilantro, chives, mint, etc.)

¼ teaspoon kosher salt

¼ teaspoon freshly ground black pepper

SERVES 4   TOTAL TIME: 15 MINUTES

1. Cook the couscous and serve: Bring the broth to a boil in a small saucepan with a tight-fitting lid. Add the couscous, stir to incorporate, then remove from the heat, cover, and let sit for 5 minutes.

2. Uncover the couscous, fluff with a fork, then stir in the olive oil, lemon juice and zest, herbs, salt, and pepper. Serve.

NUTRITIONAL INFORMATION (1 SERVING = ¾ CUP) Calories 195, Total Fat 4.2 g 6%, Saturated Fat 0.5 g 2%, Trans Fat 0.0 g, Cholesterol 0.0 mg 0%, Sodium 138.5 mg 6%, Total Carb 35.4 g 12%, Dietary Fiber 5.8 g 23%, Sugars 0.2 g, Added Sugars 0 g, Protein 6.2 g 12%, Vitamin D 0.0 mcg 0%, Calcium 28 mg 3%, Iron 1.7 mg 10%, Potassium 27.4 mg 1%

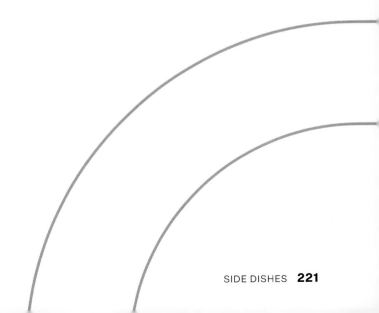

Oven-Baked Lemony Parmesan Fries

1½ pounds russet potatoes, scrubbed

Finely grated zest of 2 lemons

¼ cup olive oil

¾ teaspoon kosher salt

½ teaspoon freshly ground black pepper

5 tablespoons finely grated Parmigiano-Reggiano cheese

¼ cup finely chopped fresh parsley

We always say, here at Noom, that no food is off limits, but it's also true that traditional French fries are high in fat and calorically dense. If you're trying to improve your diet or have a weight-loss goal, you may not want to indulge in deep-fried potatoes. But with this recipe you can have your fries and eat them, too—because they aren't actually fried, making them much lower in fat and much less calorically dense.

SERVES 6 TOTAL TIME: 40 MINUTES

1. Preheat the oven to 400°F.

2. Prepare the fries: Fill a large bowl with ice water. Cut the potatoes into ½-inch planks, then cut them into ½-inch strips. Submerge the potatoes in the ice water for 5 minutes, then arrange them on clean kitchen or paper towels and pat them dry.

3. Transfer the fries to a large bowl and add all but 1 teaspoon of the zest, the olive oil, salt, and pepper. Toss to coat well. Add 4 tablespoons of the cheese and gently toss to coat again.

4. Bake and serve the fries: Arrange the fries on a rimmed baking sheet in a single layer. Sprinkle any remaining cheese mixture remaining at the bottom of the bowl over the fries. Bake until crisp and golden, 30 to 35 minutes, moving or turning the fries every 10 minutes or so to avoid sticking and to ensure even cooking and browning.

5. Transfer the fries to a large serving dish, and garnish with the remaining tablespoon cheese. Sprinkle with the parsley and reserved lemon zest and serve hot.

NUTRITIONAL INFORMATION (1 SERVING = ¾ CUP) Calories 216, Total Fat 10.9 g 17%, Saturated Fat 2.6 g 13%, Trans Fat 0.0 g, Cholesterol 5.5 mg 2%, Sodium 242.6 mg 10%, Total Carb 24.8 g 8%, Dietary Fiber 2.9 g 11%, Sugars 1.3 g, Added Sugars 0 g, Protein 5.1 g 10%, Vitamin D 0.0 mcg 0%, Calcium 92.8 mg 9%, Iron 1.4 mg 8%, Potassium 641.8 mg 18%

NOOM CHEF'S TIP: SUBMERGING POTATOES *You may wonder why recipes for baked fries often include submerging the cut potatoes in ice water. Don't skip this step! The purpose of this is to wash away some of the starch in the potatoes, which helps to make baked fries crispier.*

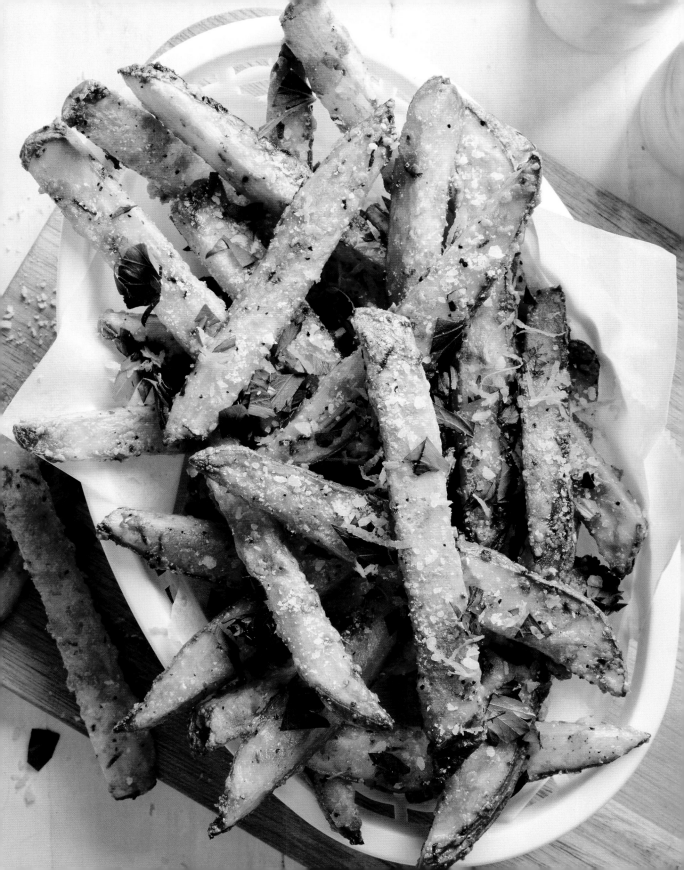

Snacks

When you're hungry—but not *too* hungry—and it's between meals, a snack is the perfect solution. But processed snacks are some of the least healthy and most caloric foods on store shelves. When you make your own, you not only get something that tastes better, you get a snack that won't derail your goals. Try these fun, colorful, unique recipes and change your snack-itude!

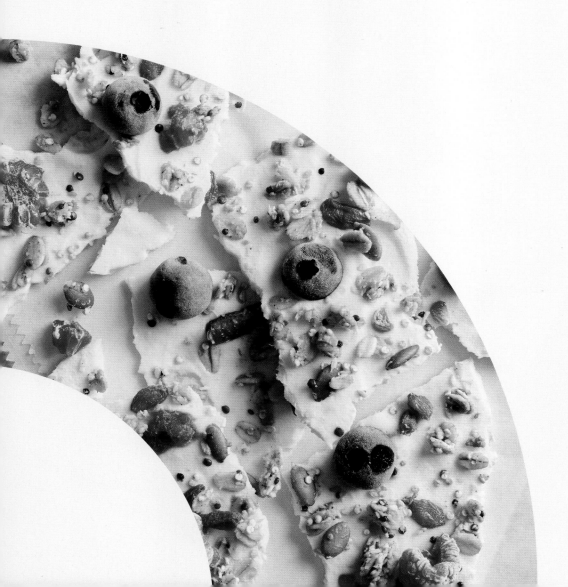

Watermelon, Mint & Blueberry Popsicles

4 cups cubed ripe seedless watermelon

10 fresh mint leaves

2 tablespoons fresh lime juice

1 tablespoon honey

1 teaspoon finely grated lime zest

1 pint fresh or frozen blueberries

You can feel good about eating—and serving—these refreshingly yummy popsicles made with real fruit and just a touch of honey. They look gorgeous and they make for a great hydrating, refreshing treat! You can buy popsicle molds in many different shapes and sizes; if you're in a real pinch, you could always just make these in ice cube trays and adjust the portioning, but we think you will love being able to make your own frozen pops!

SERVES 10   TOTAL TIME: 15 MINUTES

1. Make and freeze the popsicles: Combine the watermelon, mint, lime juice, and honey in a blender and blend until smooth, about 30 seconds. Stir in the lime zest.

2. Drop about 8 blueberries into each of 10 popsicle molds, then carefully divide the puree and pour into the molds. Freeze until solid, 4 to 5 hours.

3. Serve the popsicles: Keep these popsicles in their molds until you're ready to serve them, then gently unmold.

Note: The popsicles will keep in the freezer for up to 1 week.

NUTRITIONAL INFORMATION (1 SERVING = 1 POPSICLE) Calories 32, Total Fat 0.2 g 0%, Saturated Fat 0.1 g 0%, Trans Fat 0.0 g, Cholesterol 0.0 mg 0%, Sodium 0.9 mg 0%, Total Carb 8.2 g 3%, Dietary Fiber 0.6 g 2%, Sugars 6.7 g, Added Sugars 0 g, Protein 0.5 g 1%, Vitamin D 0.0 mcg 0%, Calcium 5.5 mg 1%, Iron 0.2 mg 1%, Potassium 82 mg 2%

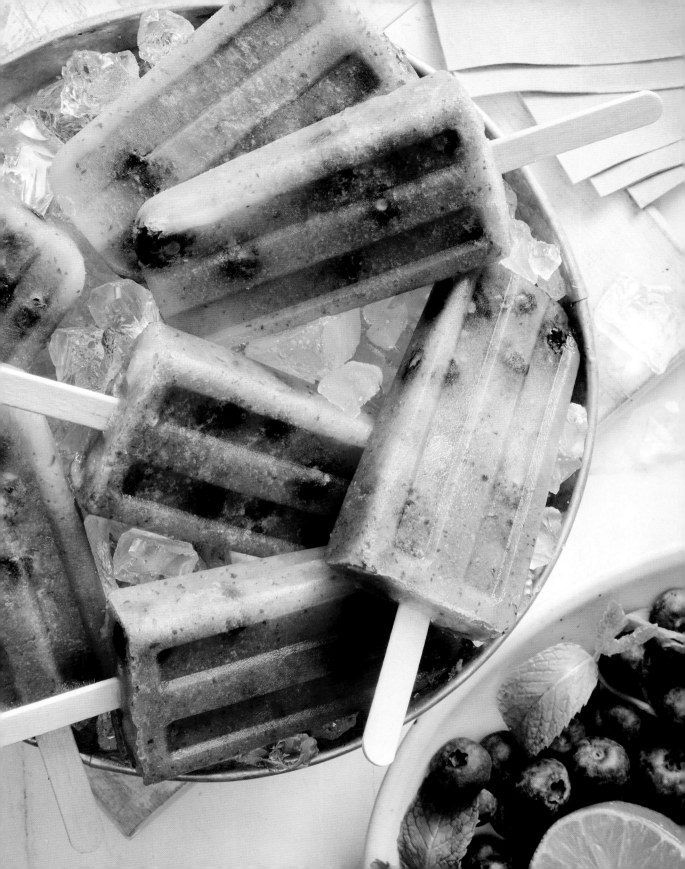

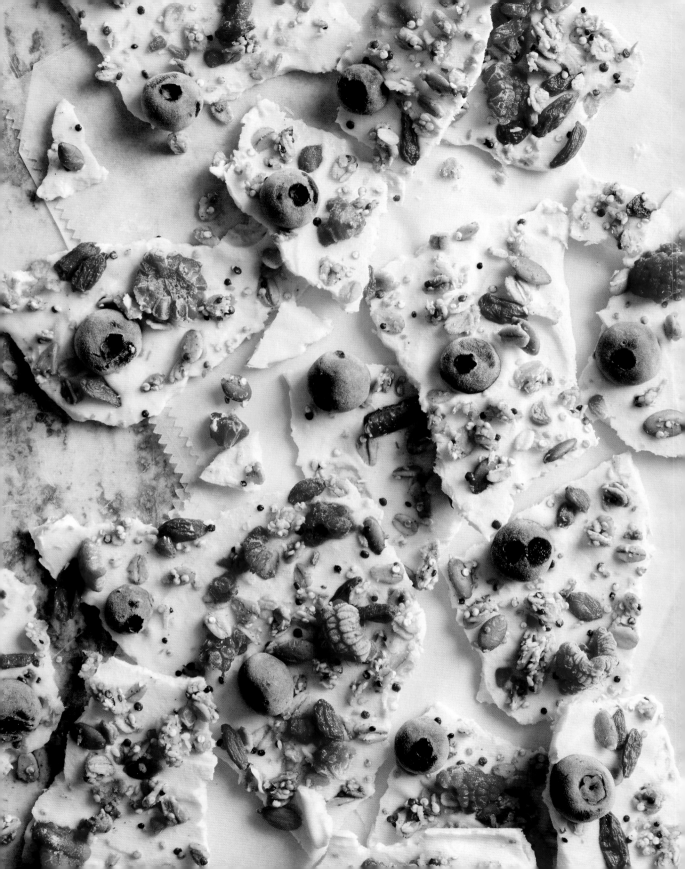

Cereal & Milk Frozen Yogurt Bark

Creamy yogurt and crunchy homemade granola combine to make a frozen yogurt bark that tastes like a candy bar but is loaded with nutritious goodness. This yogurt bark does need to remain frozen, however, so if you linger over it you may end up finishing with a spoon. Serve it in individual bowls, just in case. (It does contain cereal, after all.)

2 cups plain nonfat Greek yogurt

3 tablespoons tahini

3 tablespoons honey

1 teaspoon vanilla extract

½ cup Crispy Quinoa Granola (page 49)

¼ cup fresh or frozen blueberries

¼ cup fresh or frozen raspberries

Flaky sea salt, for garnish

SERVES 8   TOTAL TIME: 3 HOURS 10 MINUTES (INCLUDING FREEZING)

1. Mix and freeze the yogurt bark: Line a 9-by-13-inch baking pan with parchment.

2. In a medium bowl, whisk together the yogurt, tahini, 2 tablespoons of the honey, and the vanilla. Pour the mixture into the baking pan and spread it to a ¼-inch thickness.

3. Scatter the granola and then the berries over the yogurt. Drizzle with the remaining tablespoon honey and garnish with about ¾ teaspoon sea salt.

4. Freeze until the yogurt has hardened completely, at least 3 hours.

5. Break and serve the yogurt bark: Use your hands to break the frozen bark into pieces; pieces should be about 2-inch squares. Eat immediately (in frozen state).

Note: You can store the bark, in cut squares, in an airtight container in the freezer (it's okay to stack the pieces) for up to 2 weeks.

NUTRITIONAL INFORMATION (1 SERVING = 2 OR 3 PIECES) Calories 147, Total Fat 5.2 g 8%, Saturated Fat 1.2 g 6%, Trans Fat 0.1 g, Cholesterol 2.8 mg 1%, Sodium 94.5 mg 4%, Total Carb 17.9 g 6%, Dietary Fiber 1.8 g 7%, Sugars 10.1 g, Added Sugars 0 g, Protein 8.4 g 17%, Vitamin D 0.0 mcg 0%, Calcium 93.7 mg 9%, Iron 1.1 mg 6%, Potassium 160.4 mg 5%

Crispy Spiced Oven-Baked Chickpeas

Chickpeas aren't just for salads. They bake up into a delightfully crispy, flavorful snack that will leave you saying, "Popcorn who?" This recipe uses canned chickpeas, so it's fast and easy.

2 14-to-16-ounce cans chickpeas, drained and rinsed

2 tablespoons olive oil

½ teaspoon fine sea salt

1½ teaspoons smoked paprika

1½ teaspoons sweet paprika

1½ teaspoons ground cumin

SERVES 6   TOTAL TIME: 50 MINUTES

1. Preheat the oven to 425°F.

2. Dry the chickpeas: Line a rimmed baking sheet with a clean kitchen towel (or 2 layers of paper towels) and arrange the chickpeas on the towel. Place another towel on top of the chickpeas and gently shake the baking sheet to absorb any additional moisture; the drier the chickpeas are, the crisper they will get. Remove and discard any errant chickpea skins, then transfer the chickpeas to a large bowl. Remove the towel from the baking sheet.

3. Oil, season, and bake the chickpeas: Add the olive oil, salt, smoked and sweet paprikas, and cumin to the chickpeas, stir to coat, then spread them evenly on the baking sheet. Roast the chickpeas, shaking the sheet occasionally to move them around, until they are golden and crisp, 30 to 35 minutes (or longer, if necessary).

4. Cool and store the chickpeas: Allow the chickpeas to cool completely (they will crisp up further as they cool). Store the chickpeas in an airtight container for up to 4 days.

NUTRITIONAL INFORMATION (1 SERVING = ⅓ CUP) Calories 217, Total Fat 6.3 g 10%, Saturated Fat 0.9 g 4%, Trans Fat 0.0 g, Cholesterol 0.0 mg 0%, Sodium 594.9 mg 25%, Total Carb 33.7 g 11%, Dietary Fiber 6.8 g 27%, Sugars 0.2 g, Added Sugars 0 g, Protein 7.4 g 15%, Vitamin D 0.0 mcg 0%, Calcium 49.5 mg 5%, Iron 2.2 mg 12%, Potassium 278.2 mg 8%

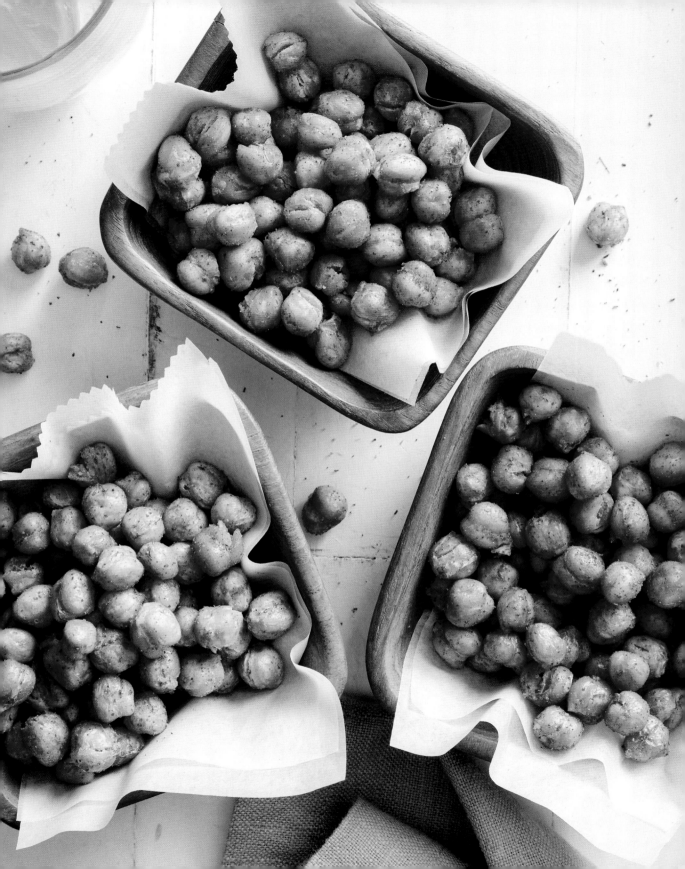

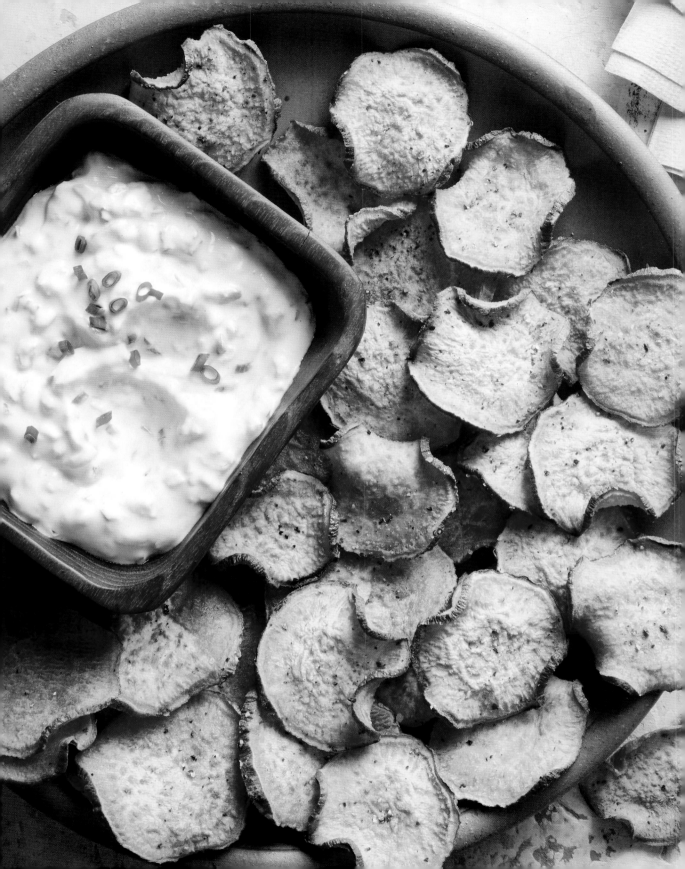

Sweet Potato Chips with Onion Dip

If you didn't make this yourself, you would never suspect just how low in fat this onion dip really is. Paired with homemade sweet potato chips, this recipe takes "chips and dip" to the next level.

FOR THE DIP

1 tablespoon olive oil

1 very large onion, finely minced (about 2 cups)

½ teaspoon kosher salt

2 garlic cloves, minced

1 cup plain nonfat Greek yogurt

2 tablespoons light mayonnaise

3 tablespoons finely minced fresh chives

1 teaspoon garlic powder

1 teaspoon onion powder

¼ teaspoon freshly ground black pepper

FOR THE CHIPS

Olive oil cooking spray

2 medium sweet potatoes (about 1 pound), scrubbed and dried, ends trimmed, peel left on

3 tablespoons olive oil

1 teaspoon kosher salt

¼ teaspoon freshly ground black pepper

SERVES 6 TOTAL TIME: 1 HOUR 45 MINUTES

1. Cook the onion: Heat the olive oil in a large (12-inch) skillet over medium-high heat. Add the onion and ¼ teaspoon of the salt and cook, stirring, for 5 minutes. Reduce the heat to medium-low, add the garlic, and cook, stirring, until the onion is golden but not charred, about 10 more minutes.

2. Transfer the onion mixture to a medium bowl; let cool for at least 10 minutes.

3. Make the dip: When the onion is no longer hot, add the yogurt, mayonnaise, chives, garlic and onion powder, remaining ¼ teaspoon salt, and the pepper and stir to combine. Chill for at least 1 hour to let the flavors meld. (Onion dip can be made up to 3 days ahead; keep covered and chilled.)

4. Make the chips: Preheat the oven to 375°F. Place a metal roasting rack on a rimmed baking sheet. Spray the rack with the olive oil cooking spray.

5. Slice the potatoes on a mandoline (see below) into thin slices (about 1⁄16 inch); if you don't have a mandoline, use your sharpest knife and cut the slices as thin as possible.

6. Pat the potatoes dry between 2 layers of paper towels, then place in a large bowl, add the olive oil, salt, and pepper, and toss, making sure the pieces aren't stuck to each other.

continued on page 234

continued from page 233

7. Separate the sweet potato slices and lay half of them on the wire rack, avoiding any overlap. Bake until golden and crisp, rotating the pan from front to back halfway through the cooking time, 25 to 30 minutes total.

8. Allow the chips to cool, then transfer to a second baking sheet or large platter. They will continue to crisp as they cool.

9. Repeat with the remaining potato slices, making sure they also bake until crisp as well.

10. Serve the chips: Place servings of the chips in individual snack cups and serve along with the dip, or place the chips in a large bowl and serve family style.

NUTRITIONAL INFORMATION (1 SERVING = ½ CUP CHIPS AND ¼ CUP DIP) Calories 199, Total Fat 10.9 g 17%, Saturated Fat 1.6 g 8%, Trans Fat 0.0 g, Cholesterol 3.6 mg 1%, Sodium 467.1 mg 19%, Total Carb 20.5 g 7%, Dietary Fiber 2.9 g 12%, Sugars 5.7 g, Added Sugars 0 g, Protein 5.6 g 11%, Vitamin D 0.0 mcg 0%, Calcium 76.4 mg 8%, Iron 0.8 mg 4%, Potassium 368.4 mg 11%

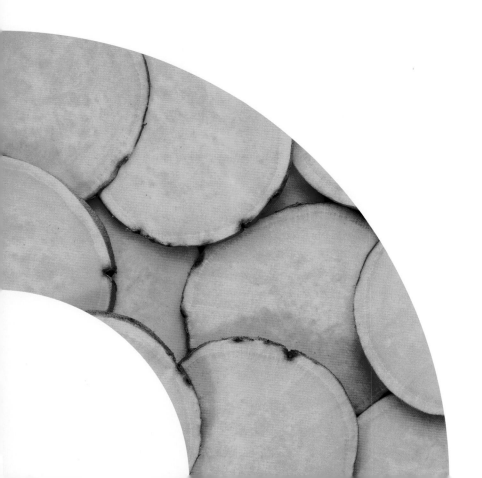

Fluffy Hummus Four Ways

1 cup cauliflower florets

¾ teaspoon fine sea salt, plus more for seasoning

1 14-to-16-ounce can chickpeas, rinsed, ¾ cup of canning liquid retained

2 tablespoons tahini

1 garlic clove

2 tablespoons fresh lemon juice, plus more for seasoning

Hummus is the perfect base for a wide variety of flavor profiles and vibrant colors. Rich in nutrients and creamy as any party dip, these recipes are surprisingly easy. We provide the base of cauliflower and hummus, then offer four variations. You might even get inspired to create further variations with your favorite flavors!

SERVES 8 TOTAL TIME: 15 MINUTES

1. Make the cauliflower: Arrange the cauliflower florets in a microwave-proof bowl, fill with 1 inch of water, and sprinkle with ¼ teaspoon of the salt. Cover with plastic wrap and microwave on high until the cauliflower is soft, 3 to 4 minutes, depending on your microwave. They should be fork-tender.

2. Make the hummus: Drain the cauliflower well, then add to a food processor along with the chickpeas, retained chickpea liquid, tahini, garlic, and remaining ½ teaspoon salt, and process until very smooth, 2 to 3 minutes.

3. Add the lemon juice and process an additional 30 seconds. Taste the hummus and season to taste with more salt and lemon juice.

4. Serve as is or choose your flavor swap: Place the hummus in a large serving bowl and serve at room temperature. Alternatively, chill first and serve cold with optional raw vegetables and/or Crispy Oat & Seed Crackers (page 240). Or, if you prefer, choose one of the following variations, blending the additional ingredients into the cauliflower-hummus mixture and then serving.

NUTRITIONAL INFORMATION(1 SERVING = ¼ CUP HUMMUS) Calories 86, Total Fat 2.6 g 4%, Saturated Fat 0.4 g 2%, Trans Fat 0.0 g, Cholesterol 0.0 mg 0%, Sodium 332.3 mg 14%, Total Carb 13.1 g 4%, Dietary Fiber 2.8 g 11%, Sugars 0.4 g, Added Sugars 0 g, Protein 3.4 g 7%, Vitamin D 0.0 mcg 0%, Calcium 35.7 mg 4%, Iron 1.1 mg 6%, Potassium 146.2 mg 4%, Flavor Swaps

continued on page 236

continued from page 235

Chipotle Hummus *(pictured)*

Into the hummus mixture, blend 2 tablespoons chopped chipotle in adobo sauce and 1 teaspoon sweet paprika; top with 1 to 2 tablespoons chopped fresh cilantro, a few jalapeño slices, and/or a sprinkling of chipotle chile powder.

NUTRITIONAL INFORMATION Calories 88, Total Fat 2.7 g 4%, Saturated Fat 0.4 g 2%, Trans Fat 0.0 g, Cholesterol 0.0 mg 0%, Sodium 349.6 mg 15%, Total Carb 13.4 g 4%, Dietary Fiber 3.1 g 12%, Sugars 0.5 g, Added Sugars 0 g, Protein 3.5 g 7%, Vitamin D 0.0 mcg 0%, Calcium 36.7 mg 4%, Iron 1.1 mg 6%, Potassium 156 mg 4%

Spice Route

Into the hummus mixture, blend 2 teaspoons garam masala. When serving, sprinkle with more garam masala and 1 tablespoon chopped fresh parsley.

NUTRITIONAL INFORMATION Calories 89, Total Fat 2.6 g 4%, Saturated Fat 0.4 g 2%, Trans Fat 0.0 g, Cholesterol 0.0 mg 0%, Sodium 333.3 mg 14%, Total Carb 13.5 g 4%, Dietary Fiber 2.8 g 11%, Sugars 0.4 g, Added Sugars 0 g, Protein 3.4 g 7%, Vitamin D 0.0 mcg 0%, Calcium 36.4 mg 4%, Iron 1.1 mg 6%, Potassium 148.8 mg 4%

Pink! *(pictured)*

SERVES 10

Into the hummus mixture, blend 1 cup chopped cooked beets, then top with ¼ cup crumbled feta, 1 or 2 tablespoons chopped fresh chives, and a sprinkling of freshly ground black pepper. (You could use canned beets, store-bought roasted beets, or your own roasted beets.)

NUTRITIONAL INFORMATION Calories 87, Total Fat 2.9 g 5%, Saturated Fat 0.9 g 4%, Trans Fat 0.0 g, Cholesterol 3.3 mg 1%, Sodium 320.8 mg 13%, Total Carb 12.4 g 4%, Dietary Fiber 2.6 g 11%, Sugars 1.8 g, Added Sugars 0 g, Protein 3.5 g 7%, Vitamin D 0.6 mcg 0%, Calcium 50.4 mg 5%, Iron 1 mg 6%, Potassium 173.2 mg 6%

Sweet Potato

SERVES 10

Into the hummus mixture, blend 1 cup diced cooked sweet potato and 1 teaspoon pumpkin pie spice; top with 2 tablespoons of Crispy Spiced Oven-Baked Chickpeas (page 230).

NUTRITIONAL INFORMATION Calories 95, Total Fat 2.4 g 4%, Saturated Fat 0.4 g 2%, Trans Fat 0.0 g, Cholesterol 0.0 mg 0%, Sodium 289.3 mg 12%, Total Carb 15.7 g 5%, Dietary Fiber 2.8 g 11%, Sugars 0.4 g, Added Sugars 0 g, Protein 3.3 g 7%, Vitamin D 0.0 mcg 0%, Calcium 38.1 mg 4%, Iron 1.1 mg 6%, Potassium 192.8 mg 6%

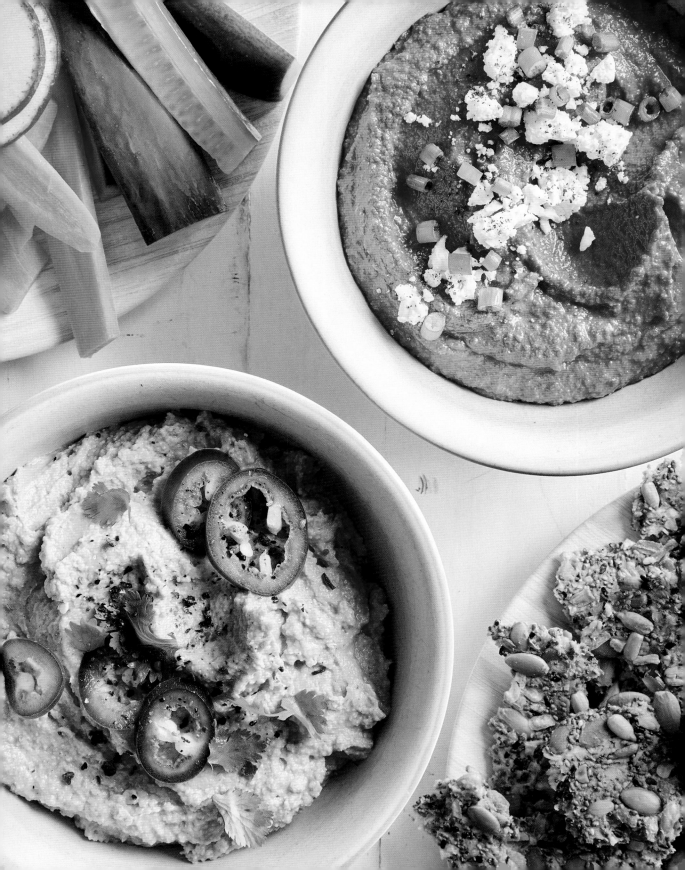

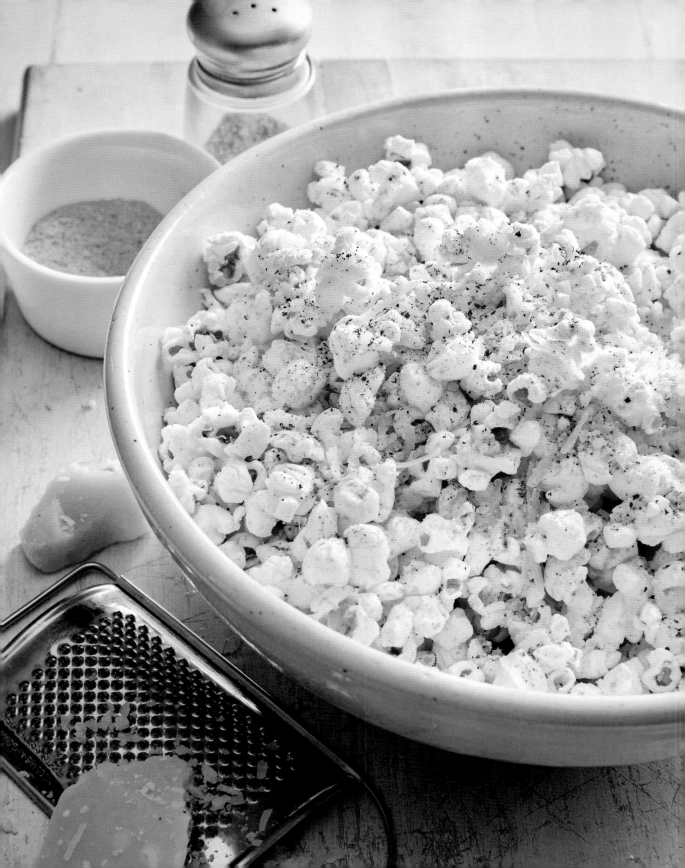

Cacio e Pepe Popcorn

1 tablespoon olive oil

¼ cup popcorn kernels

½ teaspoon fine sea salt

½ teaspoon freshly ground black pepper

½ cup finely grated Parmigiano-Reggiano cheese

1 tablespoon nutritional yeast

Cacio e pepe means "cheese and pepper" in Italian, and while this name is often applied to a classic pasta dish, we love the flavor combination in popcorn.

SERVES 6   TOTAL TIME: 15 MINUTES

1. Pop and flavor the popcorn: Heat a large (at least 6-quart) pot with a lid over high heat for 2 minutes. Add the olive oil, then add the popcorn kernels. Cover and shake the pot, keeping it directly over the grate of the stovetop, until the popcorn begins to pop.

2. Keep shaking until all the popcorn is popped, about 1½ minutes.

3. Flavor and serve the popcorn: Uncover the pot and add the salt, pepper, and cheese. Cover and shake to coat the popped corn. Let stand, covered, for 2 to 3 minutes to let the cheese melt slightly.

4. Uncover and add the nutritional yeast. Cover and shake to coat the popped corn again.

5. Transfer the flavored popcorn to a large bowl and serve.

NUTRITIONAL INFORMATION (1 SERVING = 1½ CUPS) Calories 88, Total Fat 5.3 g 8%, Saturated Fat 2.4 g 12%, Trans Fat 0.0 g, Cholesterol 8.3 mg 3%, Sodium 217 mg 9%, Total Carb 5.8 g 2%, Dietary Fiber 1.2 g 5%, Sugars 0.1 g, Added Sugars 0 g, Protein 4.4 g 9%, Vitamin D 0.0 mcg 0%, Calcium 101.2 mg 10%, Iron 0.3 mg 2%, Potassium 22 mg 1%

Crispy Oat & Seed Crackers

Crackers are fun to make, and also to break into rustic shapes. This recipe is coded orange, but only because of all the nutrient-dense seeds the crackers contain.

1 cup old-fashioned rolled oats

⅓ cup pumpkin seeds

¼ cup sunflower seeds

3 tablespoons chia seeds

3 tablespoons dried onion flakes

2 tablespoons sesame seeds

2 tablespoons poppy seeds

1 tablespoon ground flax seeds

1 tablespoon black sesame seeds

1 teaspoon kosher salt

⅔ cup boiling water

SERVES 6 TOTAL TIME: 45 MINUTES

1. Preheat the oven to 350°F.

2. Make the cracker mixture: Combine the oats, pumpkin seeds, sunflower seeds, chia seeds, onion flakes, sesame seeds, poppy seeds, flax seeds, black sesame seeds, and salt in a bowl.

3. Stir in the boiling water and let the mixture sit until it has absorbed the water and becomes firm, about 15 minutes.

4. Form the large cracker: Gather the mixture into a ball and transfer to a large sheet of parchment (the size of a large baking sheet). Form the mixture into a 6-by-8-inch rectangle, then cover with another piece of parchment.

5. Use a rolling pin to roll the dough into a thin 12-by-14-inch rectangle. Peel off and discard the top piece of parchment. Slide the dough and parchment onto a baking sheet.

6. Bake the cracker, rotating once midway through, until lightly golden and crisp, 25 to 30 minutes.

7. Serve the crackers: Let the cracker cool completely, then break into approximately 42 pieces, each about 2 inches in size.

Note: The crackers can be stored in an airtight container on the counter for up to 5 days.

NUTRITIONAL INFORMATION (1 SERVING = ½ CUP CRACKER PIECES) Calories 208, Total Fat 13.6 g 21%, Saturated Fat 1.8 g 9%, Trans Fat 0.1 g, Cholesterol 0.0 mg 0%, Sodium 253.9 mg 11%, Total Carb 16.8 g 6%, Dietary Fiber 6.5 g 26%, Sugars 1.0 g, Added Sugars 0 g, Protein 7.7 g 15%, Vitamin D 0.0 mcg 0%, Calcium 105.4 mg 11%, Iron 2.5 mg 14%, Potassium 150.9 mg 4%,

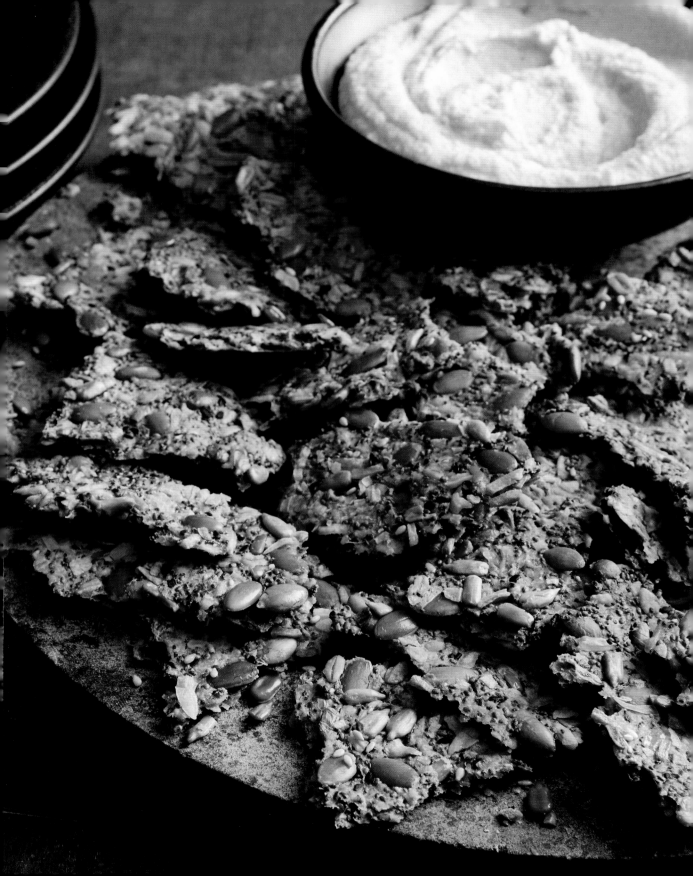

Desserts

Who says you have to skip dessert? Not us! We love a good dessert, especially when it's nutritionally—but not calorically—dense. Try these makeover recipes for dessert delight without the heavy feeling.

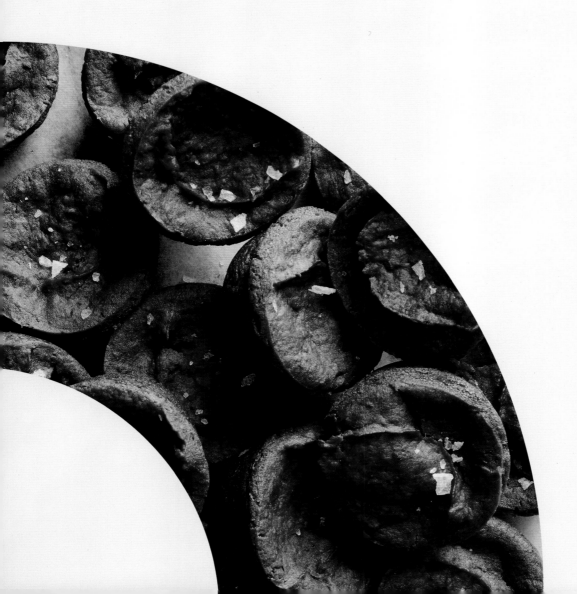

Easy Strawberry Cheesecake Ice Cream

The combination of nonfat Greek yogurt and low-fat cream cheese gives this dessert its creamy-tangy flavor, and a sprinkle of graham cracker crumbs is just enough to lend the flavor of a cheesecake crust with a fraction of the caloric density. This ice cream will keep for up to two weeks in the freezer—if you can resist!

1 cup plain nonfat Greek yogurt

¼ cup Neufchâtel (low-fat) cream cheese, softened

3 tablespoons pure maple syrup

1 teaspoon vanilla extract

½ teaspoon finely grated lemon zest

Pinch of salt

1 pound (2⅓ cups) frozen strawberries (sliced, if you can find them, for easier blending)

½ cup sliced frozen banana

2 tablespoons graham cracker crumbs

Fresh mint leaves, for garnish (optional)

SERVES 4   TOTAL TIME: 2 HOURS 10 MINUTES (INCLUDING FREEZING)

1. Make the yogurt mixture: Combine the yogurt, cream cheese, maple syrup, vanilla, lemon zest, and salt in a food processor and process until smooth. Transfer to a sandwich-sized zippered plastic bag.

2. Press out any additional air, seal, and freeze flat until almost solid, 2 to 2½ hours.

3. Finish and serve: Partially thaw the frozen strawberries and banana slices, about 5 minutes.

4. Remove the yogurt mixture from the freezer, remove it from the bag, and break it into pieces.

5. Add the pieces to the food processor. Add the strawberries and banana, and pulse the mixture to break down the fruit. Process until smooth and creamy, stopping and scraping down the sides as necessary, about 4 minutes.

6. To serve, scoop about ¾ cup into each bowl and top each bowl with 1½ teaspoons graham cracker crumbs.

Note: Alternatively, you could transfer the mixture to an airtight container (or individual serving-sized containers) and seal until ready to use (for up to 2 weeks). Defrost slightly to soften before serving.

NUTRITIONAL INFORMATION (1 SERVING = ¾ CUP, PLUS 1½ TEASPOONS CRUMBS) Calories 181, Total Fat 3.9 g 6%, Saturated Fat 2 g 10%, Trans Fat 0.0 g, Cholesterol 13.3 mg 4%, Sodium 1858 mg 77%, Total Carb 29.7 g 10%, Dietary Fiber 2.9 g 12%, Sugars 19.7 g, Added Sugars 0 g, Protein 8 g 16%, Vitamin D 0.0 mcg 0%, Calcium 114.9 mg 11%, Iron 1.3 mg 7%, Potassium 370.6 mg 11%

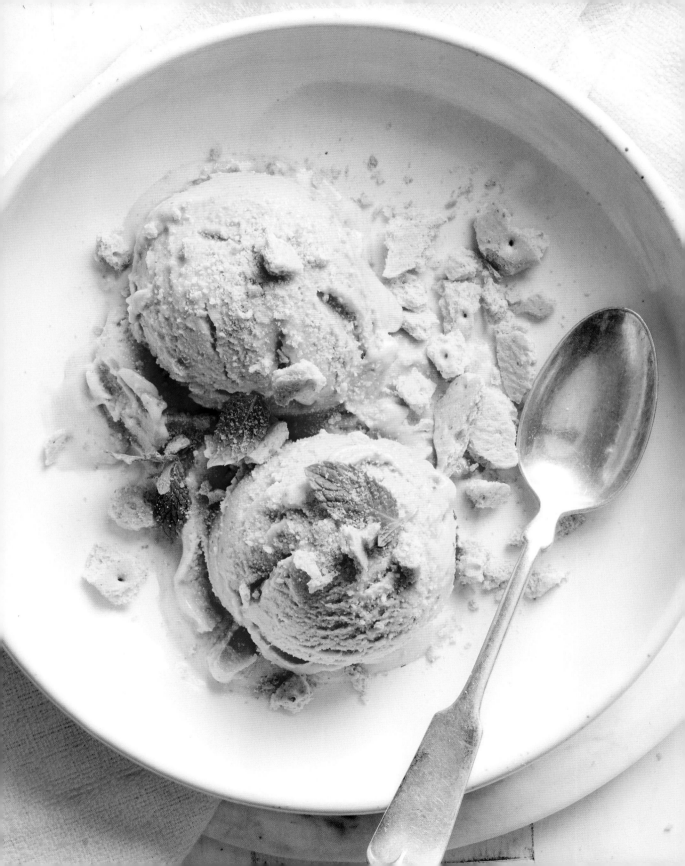

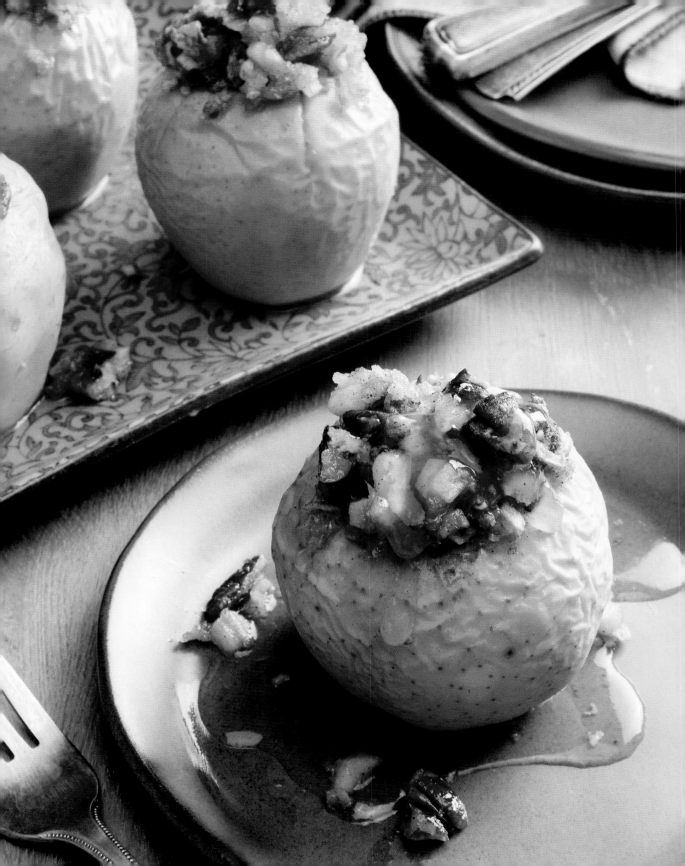

Ginger & Cinnamon Baked Apples

1 bag ginger tea

¾ cup boiling water

1 teaspoon fresh lemon juice

½ teaspoon finely grated lemon zest

3 tablespoons instant oats

2 tablespoons light brown sugar

2 tablespoons chopped toasted pecans

1 tablespoon unsalted butter, at room temperature

1 small Medjool date, pitted and chopped

1½ teaspoons grated fresh ginger (or ½ teaspoon dried ginger)

1 teaspoon ground cinnamon

7 large baking apples, such as Rome Beauty, Golden Delicious, or Jonagold

● Consider this your new favorite way to have an apple pie experience in less time and without fussy crusts. Ginger tea gives these sweet baked apples their unique flavor, and even though they are stuffed with oats, brown sugar, nuts, dates, and yes, butter, they still come out as a green food. Is it magic? When you get a taste, you'll think so!

SERVES 6 TOTAL TIME: 1 HOUR

1. Preheat the oven to 375°F.

2. Make the tea: Steep the tea in the boiling water for 5 to 10 minutes. Let cool to room temperature.

3. Make the filling: To a medium bowl, add the lemon juice and zest, then add the oats, brown sugar, pecans, butter, date, ginger, and cinnamon. Stir to combine.

4. Prepare the apples: Peel, core, and very finely chop 1 apple. Add it to the filling mixture.

5. Use an apple corer or paring knife to remove the cores from the remaining 6 apples, leaving the bottom 1 inch of the apples intact. Use a paring knife to widen the space left by the core so you have about a 1-inch circle in the center of each apple.

6. Stuff and bake the apples: Stuff each apple with 2 to 3 tablespoons of the filling, packing any extra filling around the top, then arrange the stuffed apples in a 9- or 10-inch glass baking dish. Pour the tea around the apples (but not on top of the filling), seal the dish tightly with foil, and bake until the apples are tender but not mushy, about 25 minutes. Uncover the apples, then bake until the topping is golden and crisp, an additional 10 minutes.

7. Serve the apples: Let the apples cool slightly, then place in 6 individual bowls, drizzling the liquid from the baking dish over the apples.

NUTRITIONAL INFORMATION (1 SERVING = 1 STUFFED APPLE) Calories 194, Total Fat 4.7 g 7%, Saturated Fat 2.2 g 11%, Trans Fat 0.1 g, Cholesterol 5.1 mg 2%, Sodium 27.7 mg 1%, Total Carb 42.9 g 14%, Dietary Fiber 7 g 28%, Sugars 32.2 g, Added Sugars 0 g, Protein 1.6 g 3%, Vitamin D 1.4 mcg 0%, Calcium 31.7 mg 3%, Iron 0.6 mg 3%, Potassium 320.3 mg 9%

Thai Mango & Coconut Delight

Is mango the best of all fruits? You could probably convince us, especially when fresh, juicy mango slices are drizzled with coconut cream sauce and sprinkled with puffed rice, peanuts, and fresh mint. Simple, easy, and delightful, indeed.

2 tablespoons unsweetened canned coconut milk (stir before measuring)

2 teaspoons light brown sugar

⅛ teaspoon fine sea salt, such as Maldon

1 large mango (¾ pound), peeled, pitted, and thinly sliced

2 tablespoons puffed rice cereal

1 tablespoon chopped salted peanuts

1 tablespoon chopped fresh mint

SERVES 4 TOTAL TIME: 10 MINUTES

1. Prepare the sauce: Whisk the coconut milk, brown sugar, and salt in a small bowl until the sugar and salt are dissolved. (To make a smoother sauce, microwave it for 30 seconds to melt the coconut solids.)

2. Serve the mango: Arrange the sliced mango on 4 dessert plates. Drizzle the sauce evenly over the slices, then sprinkle with the puffed rice, peanuts, and mint and serve.

NUTRITIONAL INFORMATION (1 SERVING = ¼ MANGO, PLUS SCANT TABLESPOON SAUCE AND SPRINKLE OF TOPPING) Calories 100, Total Fat 2.9 g 4%, Saturated Fat 1.6 g 8%, Trans Fat 0.0 g, Cholesterol 0.0 mg 0%, Sodium 75.4 mg 3%, Total Carb 19.2 g 6%, Dietary Fiber 1.9 g 8%, Sugars 16.8 g, Added Sugars 0 g, Protein 1.5 g 3%, Vitamin D 0.0 mcg 0%, Calcium 15.9 mg 2%, Iron 0.7 mg 3%, Potassium 218.8 mg 6%

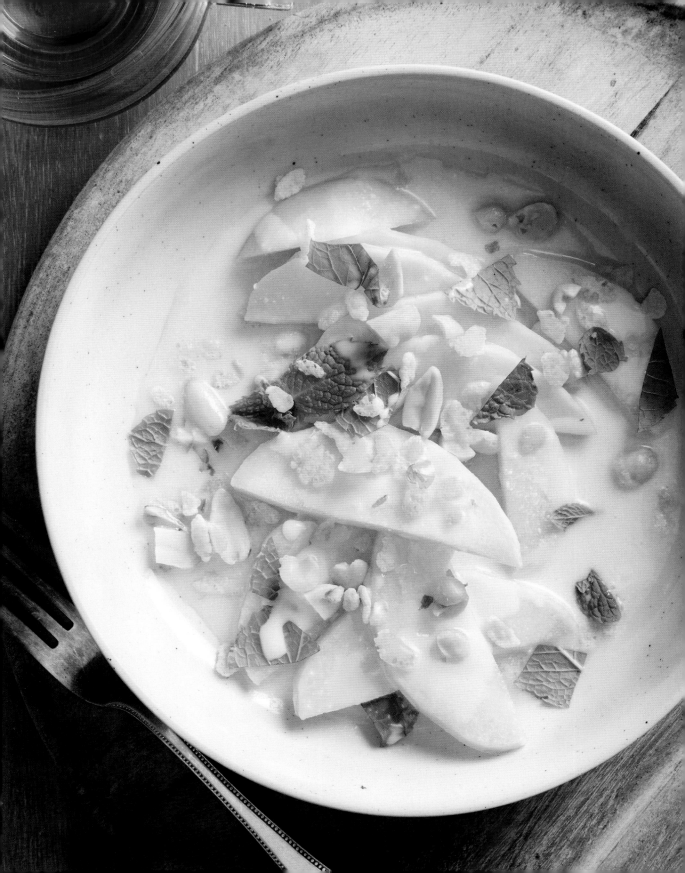

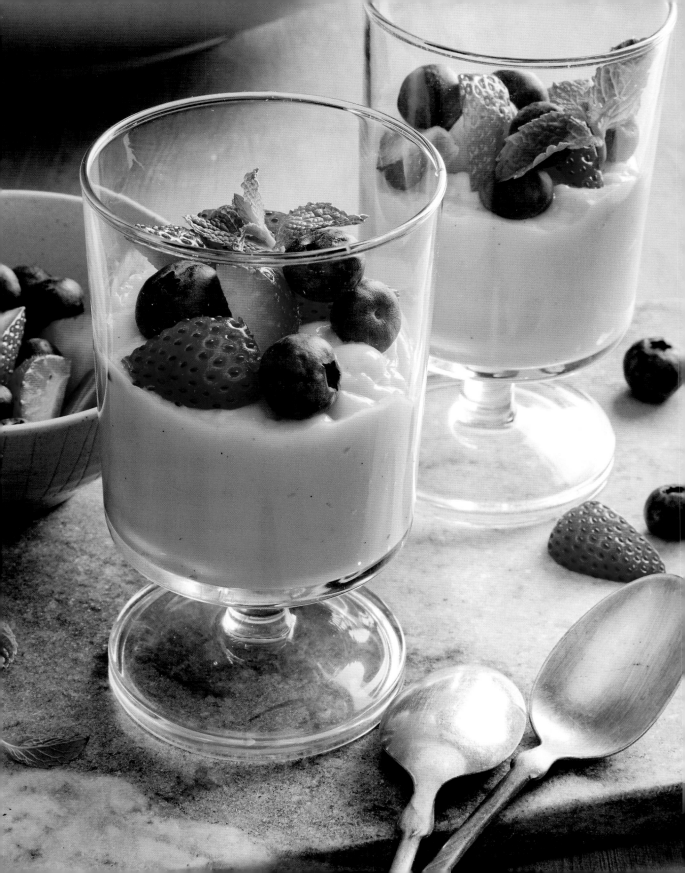

Vanilla
Pudding

2 cups 2 percent milk, cold

3 tablespoons cornstarch

¼ cup pure maple syrup

2 large egg yolks

Seeds scraped from 1 vanilla
bean (or 1 teaspoon vanilla
extract)

⅛ teaspoon kosher salt

½ cup fresh berries of choice,
sliced if large

Fresh mint leaves, for garnish

This creamy vanilla pudding is naturally sweetened with maple syrup, and the fresh, jewel-like berries add significant nutritional benefits. Use whatever berries are in season.

SERVES 4 TOTAL TIME: 3 HOURS 12 MINUTES (INCLUDING CHILLING)

1. Mix and cook the pudding: Set a fine-mesh sieve over a bowl.

2. In a small saucepan, whisk together the milk and cornstarch, then whisk in maple syrup and egg yolks until blended.

3. Place the saucepan over medium heat and bring to a boil, whisking constantly, until the pudding thickens and bubbles and the whisk leaves a distinct impression when lifted from the mixture, 4 to 5 minutes.

4. Gently pour the pudding through the strainer, pressing through gently.

5. Whisk in the vanilla seeds and the salt and cool, stirring often, for 10 minutes.

6. Press a piece of plastic wrap over the top of the pudding to prevent a skin from forming. (Or divide among 4 serving bowls and cover individually.)

7. Refrigerate until chilled and less jiggly but still creamy and a little loose, about 3 hours.

8. Serve the pudding: Remove the plastic wrap from the pudding. Divide the pudding among 4 serving bowls (if you haven't already) and top each serving with 2 tablespoons of the berries. Garnish with the mint leaves and serve.

NUTRITIONAL INFORMATION (1 SERVING = ½ CUP PUDDING AND 2 TABLESPOONS BERRIES) Calories 177, Total Fat 4.7 g 7%, Saturated Fat 2.3 g 11%, Trans Fat 0.0 g, Cholesterol 101.5 mg 34%, Sodium 115.3 mg 5%, Total Carb 27.7 g 9%, Dietary Fiber 0.5 g 2%, Sugars 13.9 g, Added Sugars 0 g, Protein 5.7 g 11%, Vitamin D 18.5 mcg 5%, Calcium 182.9 mg 18%, Iron 0.4 mg 2%, Potassium 257.8 mg 7%

NOOM CHEF'S TIP: USING VANILLA BEANS *Vanilla extract is a nice and easy way to add vanilla flavor to your recipes, but nothing beats the flavor of a real vanilla bean. If you decide to try one in this recipe (or any other), use a sharp knife to split the vanilla bean from top to bottom, then scrape out the seeds with the knife (use the seeds in the recipe and discard the pods).*

Vietnamese Iced Coffee Granita

2½ cups strong brewed coffee, at room temperature

½ cup unsweetened vanilla almond milk

2½ tablespoons pure maple syrup

1 teaspoon vanilla extract

½ teaspoon ground cinnamon

⅛ teaspoon fine sea salt

3 tablespoons sweetened condensed milk

Icy coffee granita, drizzled with sweetened condensed milk, tastes like a decadent dessert, but it's actually a light and refreshing drink—and it's a green food! Hooray for "green" desserts! This treat tastes like an icy coffee-flavored frappe, but you can make it at home, with less sugar. Just remember that it still has caffeine, so don't have it too close to bedtime!

SERVES 6 TOTAL TIME: 3 HOURS (INCLUDING FREEZING)

1. Mix the granita: In a 4-cup or larger bowl with a spout for pouring, combine the coffee, almond milk, maple syrup, vanilla, cinnamon, and salt.

2. Pour the mixture into a 2- to 3-quart baking dish or a 9-by-13-inch baking pan.

3. Freeze the granita: Make room in your freezer for your baking dish. Put the pan with the coffee mixture into the freezer to chill. Set a timer for 30 minutes.

4. Remove the pan from the freezer. Scrape every 30 minutes. For a photo and detailed instructions, see page 28.

5. Serve the granita: Divide the granita among 6 serving bowls or glasses and drizzle each bowl with 1½ teaspoons of the sweetened condensed milk. Serve immediately.

Note: You can store leftover granita in the freezer. You may need to scrape and break it apart again before serving.

NUTRITIONAL INFORMATION (1 SERVING = 1 CUP GRANITA, PLUS 1½ TEASPOONS CONDENSED MILK) Calories 63, Total Fat 1.1 g 2%, Saturated Fat 0.6 g 3%, Trans Fat 0.0 g, Cholesterol 3.2 mg 1%, Sodium 66.7 mg 3%, Total Carb 12.4 g 4%, Dietary Fiber 0.2 g 1%, Sugars 11.6 g, Added Sugars 0 g, Protein 1.0 g 2%, Vitamin D 0.6 mcg 0%, Calcium 65 mg 6%, Iron 0.1 mg 0%, Potassium 1.1 mg 2%

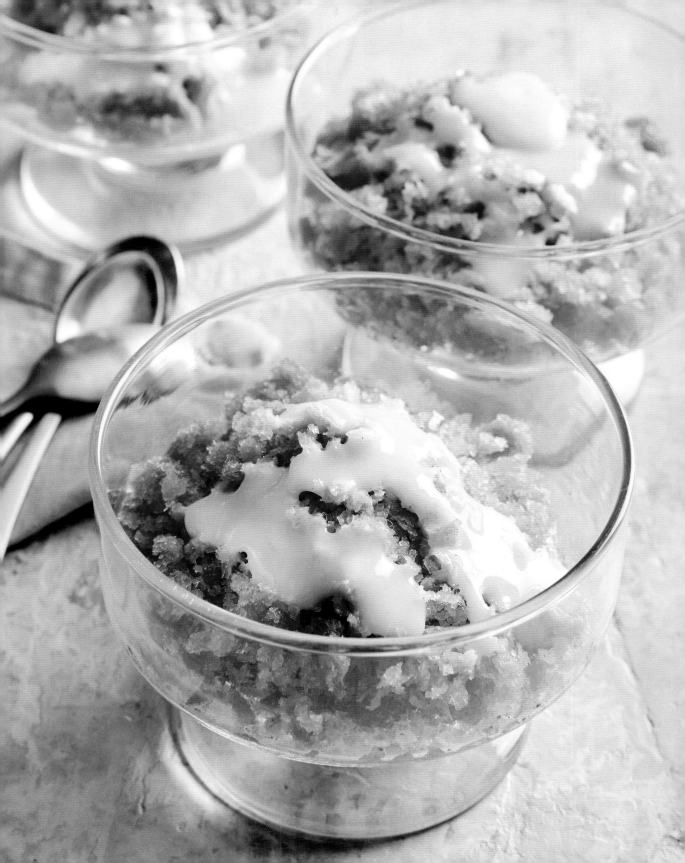

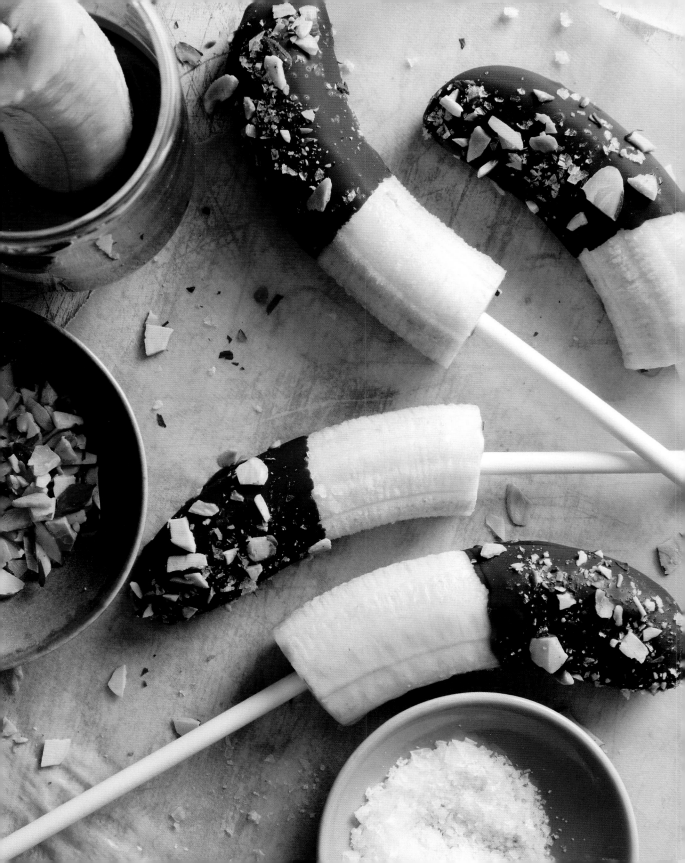

Dark Chocolate Banana Pops

4 ripe (but not soft) large bananas

4 ounces bittersweet chocolate chips or chunks

2 teaspoons coconut oil

2 tablespoons finely chopped salted roasted almonds

1 teaspoon flaky sea salt, such as Maldon

No kidding: this recipe is as decadent as any ice cream bar, but it's packed with nutrients. What a great alternative! These pops will last in the freezer for two weeks when you wrap them properly, so you can make a whole batch at the same time. Bananas, you complete us.

SERVES 8 TOTAL TIME: 2 HOURS 10 MINUTES

1. Prep and freeze the bananas: Cut the bananas in half crosswise. Skewer a popsicle stick into each half.

2. Line a plate or baking sheet with wax paper, arrange the bananas on the plate, and freeze until solid, 2 to 3 hours.

3. Make the chocolate and dip the pops: Place the chocolate and coconut oil in a small microwavable bowl and microwave until melted, about 60 seconds, stopping and stirring every 15 to 20 seconds. Using a rubber scraper, transfer the melted chocolate to a tall narrow glass.

4. Remove the bananas from the freezer and dip each halfway into the chocolate, then lift it out, letting the excess drip off.

5. Quickly sprinkle with a few almonds and some salt, rotating so both sides of the pop are covered (the last pops may be a bit messier). The chocolate will harden almost immediately.

6. Arrange the pops on the plate, with room between them, and refreeze for 15 minutes.

7. Serve the pops: Serve 1 frozen pop per person.

Note: To freeze the pops for later, individually wrap them in wax paper and store in the freezer for up to 2 weeks.

NUTRITIONAL INFORMATION (1 SERVING = 1 POP) Calories 151, Total Fat 7.2 g 11%, Saturated Fat 4.5 g 22%, Trans Fat 0.0 g, Cholesterol 0.0 mg 0%, Sodium 241.9 mg 10%, Total Carb 21.5 g 7%, Dietary Fiber 2.7 g 11%, Sugars 12.1 g, Added Sugars 0 g, Protein 2 g 4%, Vitamin D 0.0 mcg 0%, Calcium 8.7 mg 1%, Iron 0.6 mg 3%, Potassium 226.6 mg 6%

Fudgy Two-Bite Brownies

6 ounces peeled and cubed raw sweet potato

1½ ounces dark chocolate (at least 70 percent cacao), chopped

1 cup black beans, drained and rinsed, then drained again

¼ cup coconut oil

¼ cup white whole wheat or rice flour

3 tablespoons unsweetened plain or vanilla almond milk

3 tablespoons lightly packed dark brown sugar

2 tablespoons granulated sugar

2 tablespoons unsweetened cocoa powder

2 teaspoons vanilla extract

½ teaspoon baking powder

⅛ teaspoon fine sea salt

Flaky sea salt, for garnish

Once these brownies have cooled completely you really can't even taste the secret ingredients, but if you dig in while they're still warm you might get some hints of the beans. It's not bad, but they'll be more chocolatey if you can resist them straight out of the oven (the struggle is real)!

SERVES 12 TOTAL TIME: 1 HOUR (INCLUDING COOLING)

1. Prepare the sweet potato: Preheat the oven to 375°F. Lightly coat 24 cups of a mini muffin tin with cooking spray.

2. Place the sweet potato in a small saucepan, add about 1 inch of water, bring to a boil over high heat, cover, reduce the heat to low, and simmer until the sweet potato is tender, 12 to 13 minutes.

3. Drain well, cool, then mash into a paste (you should have about 1 cup).

4. Prepare the brownie batter: Place the chocolate in a small bowl and microwave on high, stopping to stir every 30 seconds, until melted and smooth, about 1 minute 30 seconds.

5. Add the mashed sweet potato and melted chocolate to a food processor along with the beans, coconut oil, flour, almond milk, brown sugar, granulated sugar, cocoa powder, vanilla, baking powder, and salt. Process, stopping and scraping down the sides of the processor bowl if necessary, until very smooth, 30 to 45 seconds.

6. Bake and serve the brownies: Using about 1 generous tablespoon batter for each brownie, evenly divide the batter among the muffin cups and bake until the tops are crackled and shiny, 30 to 35 minutes.

7. Move the pan to a wire rack and cool completely to allow the centers to set before releasing them from the tin, about 30 minutes.

8. Garnish the brownies with the flaky sea salt, if desired, and serve at room temperature, or refrigerate and serve later.

Note: These brownies will keep, in a sealed container, in the refrigerator for up to 4 days.

NUTRITIONAL INFORMATION (1 SERVING = 2 BROWNIE BITES) Calories 118, Total Fat 6.3 g 10%, Saturated Fat 4.9 g 25%, Trans Fat 0.0 g, Cholesterol 0.0 mg 0%, Sodium 122.5 mg 5%, Total Carb 14.8 g 5%, Dietary Fiber 2.6 g 10%, Sugars 6 g, Added Sugars 0 g, Protein 2.3 g 5%, Vitamin D 0.0 mcg 0%, Calcium 35.9 mg 4%, Iron 1.0 mg 5%, Potassium 132.8 mg 4%

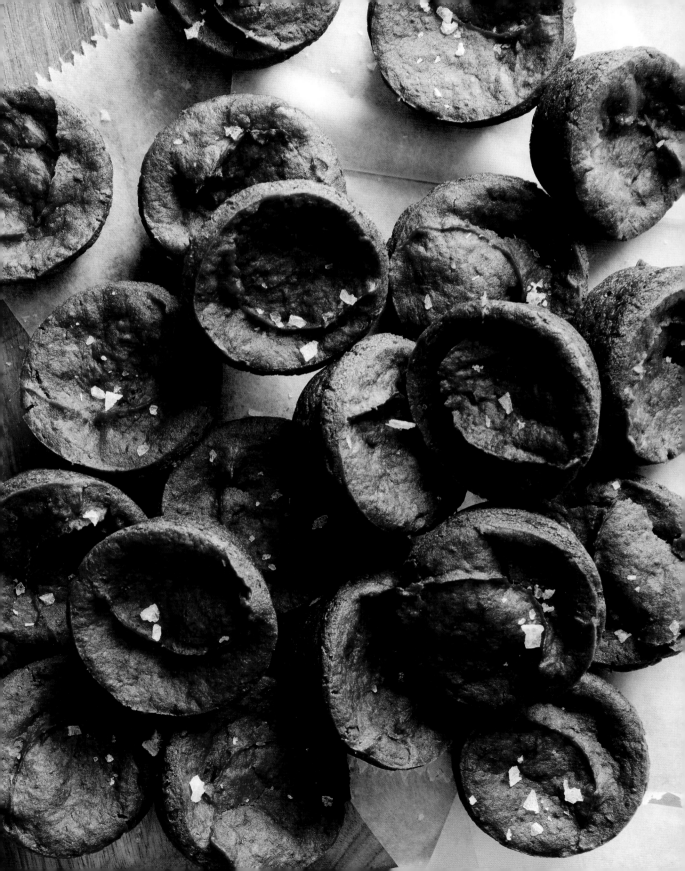

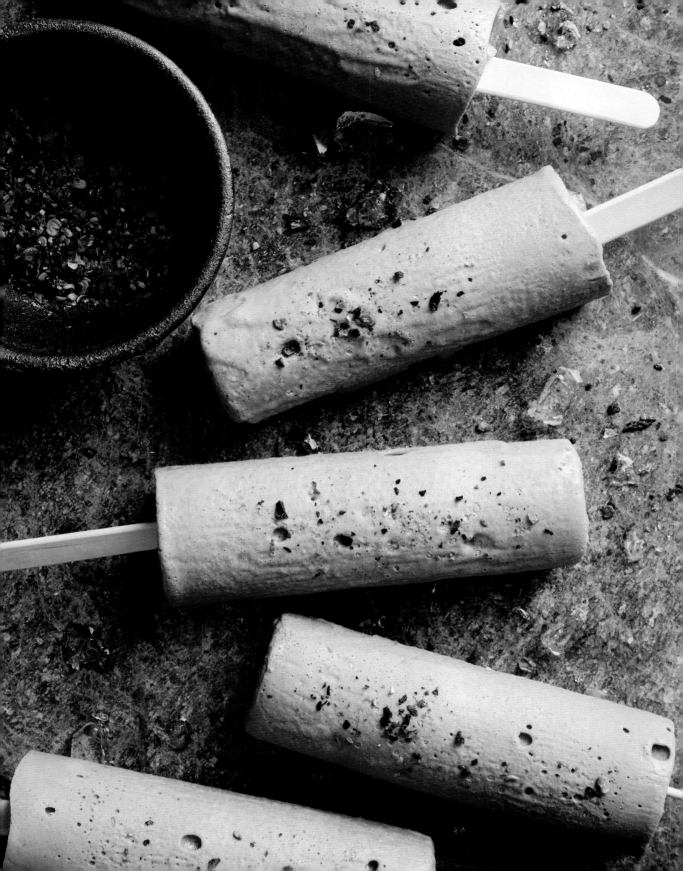

Mexican Hot Chocolate Fudge Pops

These fudge pops are infused with protein from the silken tofu and egg whites. Flavored with cinnamon and cayenne (just a hint for a little warmth), these are the perfect dessert or snack for when a chocolate craving hits.

1 12-ounce block silken tofu

2 ounces high-quality bittersweet chocolate, finely chopped

5 tablespoons confectioners' sugar

2 tablespoons unsweetened cocoa powder

2 teaspoons vanilla extract

½ teaspoon ground cinnamon

⅛ teaspoon cayenne (optional)

⅛ teaspoon fine sea salt, such as Maldon

2 large egg whites (or equivalent meringue powder if avoiding raw eggs)

Pinch of cream of tartar

Red pepper flakes or chili powder

MAKES 8 POPS TOTAL TIME: 3 HOURS 20 MINUTES

1. Drain the tofu: Carefully transfer the tofu to a fine-mesh strainer and drain well.

2. Melt the chocolate: Microwave the chocolate in a small microwave-safe bowl on high power, stopping and stirring every 15 to 20 seconds, until the chocolate is melted and smooth, about 90 seconds. Let cool.

3. Mix the pudding: Transfer the tofu to the small bowl of a food processor. Add the confectioners' sugar, cocoa powder, vanilla, cinnamon, cayenne, and salt. Process the mixture, stopping the processor to scrape down the sides of the bowl if necessary, until smooth, about 1½ minutes.

4. Add the melted chocolate and blend until smooth, about 15 seconds. Transfer to a large bowl.

5. Form the pudding pops and freeze: In a medium bowl, whisk the egg whites and cream of tartar until firm peaks form, 2 to 3 minutes (easiest done with an electric mixer). Gently fold the egg whites into the chocolate mixture.

6. Divide the pudding among 8 popsicle molds. Use a table knife to remove any large air bubbles. Top off the molds with any remaining chocolate mixture. Tap the molds on the counter to remove any remaining air bubbles. Place popsicle sticks in the molds. Freeze until solid, about 3 hours, or up to 2 weeks.

7. Serve the pops: To serve, run the molds under hot water for 5 seconds to release the popsicles. Dust the popsicles with the red pepper flakes and serve immediately.

Note: Consuming raw or undercooked eggs may increase the risk of foodborne illness.

NUTRITIONAL INFORMATION (1 SERVING = 1 POP) Calories 92, Total Fat 4.2 g 6%, Saturated Fat 1.9 g 10%, Trans Fat 0.0 g, Cholesterol 0.0 mg 0%, Sodium 45.6 mg 2%, Total Carb 11.2 g 4%, Dietary Fiber 1.1 g 4%, Sugars 8.5 g, Added Sugars 0 g, Protein 3.7 g 7%, Vitamin D 0.0 mcg 0%, Calcium 17.3 mg 2%, Iron 1.1 mg 6%, Potassium 117.4 mg 3%

Rice-Wrapper Banana Loti

1 tablespoon coconut oil

2 large egg whites, lightly beaten

4 8-inch round rice paper wrappers

2 large ripe bananas, cut into ½-inch slices

4 teaspoons sweetened condensed milk

8 teaspoons chopped salted cashews

Chopped fresh mint, for garnish

Bananas are packed with nutrients and are an easy, on-the-go breakfast or snack. Banana loti is a popular street food in Thailand, and it consists of bananas wrapped in rice paper that have been fried and drizzled with sweetened condensed milk. This version uses very little oil and has just a drizzle of the sweet stuff. Dessert should always be this delicious and nutritious!

SERVES 4   TOTAL TIME: 15 MINUTES

1. Preheat the oven to 200°F. Place a small baking pan or baking sheet in the oven.

2. Place a medium (9- or 10-inch) nonstick skillet over medium heat. Brush lightly with about 1 teaspoon of the coconut oil.

3. Moisten the rice paper: Put the egg whites in a wide plate with sides or a small 9- or 10-inch rimmed tray and whisk again lightly. Dip a wrapper briefly into the egg whites, then flip it to coat both sides. Let it sit in the egg whites just briefly, until it becomes flexible.

4. Transfer the wrapper to a cutting board or cookie sheet. Repeat with remaining 3 wrappers.

5. Assemble the loti: See photos and instructions on page 28.

6. Cook the loti: Using a spatula, carefully place a filled wrapper into the hot skillet. Cook the loti until the underside is crisped and golden spots appear, 1 to 2 minutes. Carefully flip over and cook until the other side is crisped, another 1 to 2 minutes. Transfer to the baking dish in the oven to keep warm.

7. Repeat, frying the remaining 3 loti.

8. Serve the loti: Put the cooked loti on a large serving platter Drizzle each with 1 teaspoon of the condensed milk, then top each with 2 teaspoons of the cashews. Garnish with mint and serve immediately.

NUTRITIONAL INFORMATION (1 SERVING = 1 LOTI, WITH TOPPINGS) Calories 174, Total Fat 6.8 g 11%, Saturated Fat 3.9 g 19%, Trans Fat 0.0 g, Cholesterol 2.2 mg 1%, Sodium 157.7 mg 7%, Total Carb 25.4 g 8%, Dietary Fiber 1.7 g 7%, Sugars 11.1 g, Added Sugars 0 g, Protein 4.3 g 9%, Vitamin D 0.4 mcg 0%, Calcium 24.8 mg 2%, Iron 0.6 mg 3%, Potassium 294.1 mg 8%

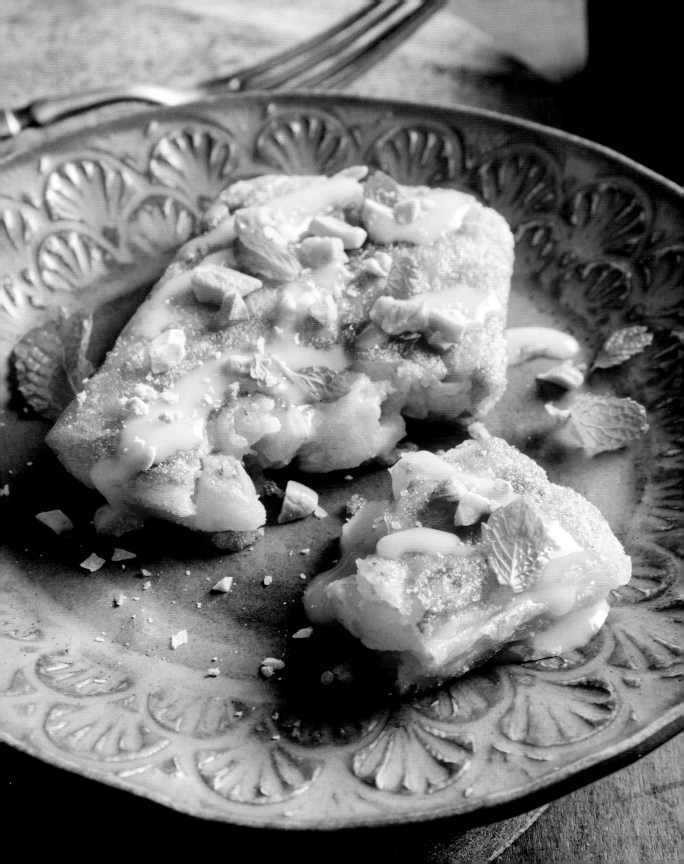

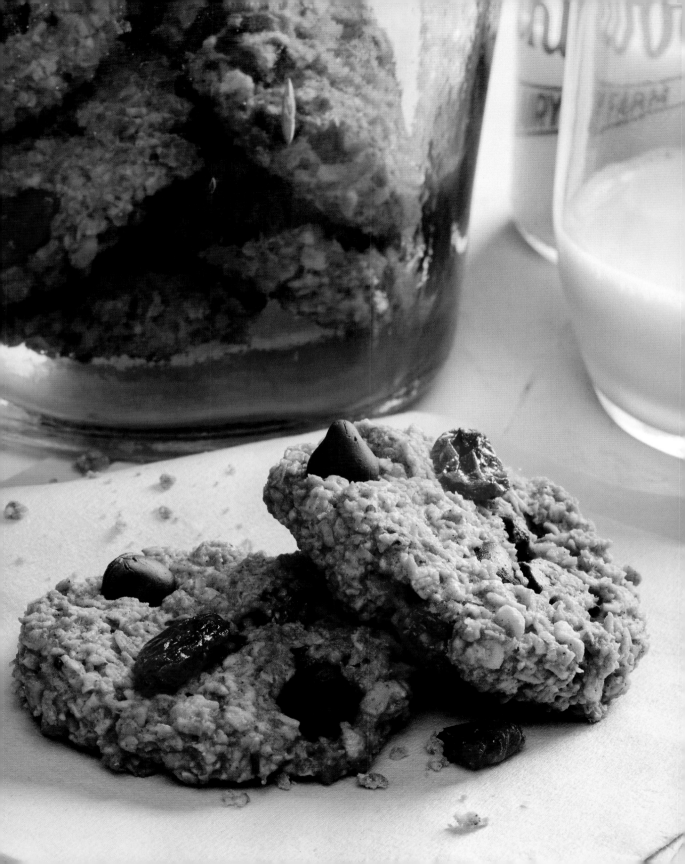

Oatmeal-Raisin Chocolate Chip Cookies

⅓ cup demerara sugar

2 tablespoons natural-style chunky peanut butter or almond butter

1 tablespoon unsalted butter, softened

2 cups quick-cooking oats

¼ cup applesauce

3 tablespoons all-purpose flour

1 large egg, lightly beaten

1 teaspoon ground cinnamon

1 teaspoon vanilla extract

¼ teaspoon fine sea salt

¼ cup semisweet chocolate chips

¼ cup golden raisins

Here's the secret to enjoying cookies while focusing on moderation: make them small. These cute-as-a-button oatmeal-raisin chocolate chip cookies contain demerara sugar, a partially refined sugar that still contains some of its minerals, plus golden raisins that stand in for half the chocolate chips without replacing them entirely. Sweet!

SERVES 12 TOTAL TIME: 50 MINUTES (INCLUDING CHILLING)

1. Make the cookie dough: Combine the demerara sugar, peanut butter, and butter in the bowl of a stand mixer fitted with a paddle attachment (or in a mixing bowl using a hand mixer) and beat on medium speed until light and slightly fluffy, 1 to 2 minutes.

2. Add the oats, applesauce, flour, egg, cinnamon, vanilla, and salt, and beat until just incorporated, about 30 seconds. Fold in the chocolate chips and raisins.

3. Cover the bowl with plastic wrap and place in the refrigerator to chill for 30 minutes.

4. Form and bake the cookies: Preheat the oven to 350°F. Line 2 baking sheets with parchment.

5. Roll one tablespoon of dough at a time into a ball. Place the balls on the baking sheet 1½ inches apart (they won't spread when they bake). Flatten each ball and make an indentation in the middle using the back of a fork.

6. Bake the cookies until the edges and tops are golden, 10 to 12 minutes, reversing the baking sheets halfway through.

7. Let the cookies cool slightly on the sheets before transferring them to a cooling rack.

8. Serve the cookies: Arrange 2 cookies on each plate and serve while still warm or at room temperature.

Note: Cookies can be cooled and placed in a cookie jar on the counter; they will stay fresh for up to 2 days, or freeze for up to 2 weeks.

NUTRITIONAL INFORMATION (1 SERVING = 2 COOKIES) Calories 143, Total Fat 5 g 8%, Saturated Fat 2 g 10%, Trans Fat 0.1 g, Cholesterol 18 mg 6%, Sodium 53.1 mg 2%, Total Carb 23.1 g 8%, Dietary Fiber 2.1 g 8%, Sugars 10.8 g, Added Sugars 0 g, Protein 3.6 g 7%, Vitamin D 4.1 mcg 1%, Calcium 14.9 mg 1%, Iron 1.1 mg 6%, Potassium 83.6 mg 2%

Acknowledgments

A book like *The Noom Kitchen* is truly a collaboration. So many people contributed to making this book all that it is that it would be difficult to name them all—but we have a can-do spirit here at Noom, so we're going to try!

First and foremost, we must thank our founders, Artem Petakov and Saeju Jeong, whose creativity, mutual drive to change the world for the better, and entrepreneurial spirit are responsible for Noom's existence and continued growth. A very special thanks to our Noom coaches, who work tirelessly one-on-one to help our Noomers succeed and whose compassion and skill have been integral to the making of this book. Many others on the Noom team have contributed their time, sweat, and tears—especially Jackson Tilley, who was the linchpin for this second Noom book. His clear-eyed vision and cheerful collaborative spirit made this book possible. Thanks are also due to many members of various Noom teams—especially Melissa Rubenstein, Sabrina Ling, Tina Finkelstein, Sarah Parkinson, Sneha Keshwan, Beth Downey, and Ioana Tabra.

Adeena Sussman captured the global palette of Noomers around the world through her innovative, delicious recipe development. Her skill in the kitchen is matched only by her skill on the page, and for her work on this book we are eternally grateful. Thanks to Eve Adamson, whose knack for capturing Noom's voice gave this book its tone and structure, and for being so quick and easy to work with. Thanks also to the whole team at Waterbury for their time and effort in bringing these pages to life.

We thank everyone at Simon Element, especially Leah Miller, our benevolent leader. Thanks to publisher extraordinaire Richard Rhorer, Nicole Bond, Jessie McNiel, Patrick Sullivan for the fabulous cover, Jessica Preeg, Elizabeth Breeden, and the countless other people who worked hard to make this book a reality. Thanks to the entire team at CAA, especially Cindy Uh, for brilliantly connecting all the working parts, and Jamie Stockton, for moving the project forward.

And finally, thanks to *you*. Whether you've been with us for a while or are just joining us, you and your journey are Noom's reason for being.

Notes

WELCOME TO NOOM'S FIRST EVER COOKBOOK

1. Simon N. Thornton, "Increased Hydration Can Be Associated with Weight Loss," *Frontiers in Nutrition* 3, no. 18 (June 2016), https://www.ncbi.nlm.nih.gov/pmc/articles/PMC4901052/.

2. Derek C. Miketinas et al., "Fiber Intake Predicts Weight Loss and Dietary Adherence in Adults Consuming Calorie-Restricted Diets: The POUNDS Lost (Preventing Overweight Using Novel Dietary Strategies) Study," *Journal of Nutrition* 149, no. 10 (October 2019): 1742–48, https://doi.org/10.1093/jn/nxz117.

3. Peter Cronin et al., "Dietary Fibre Modulates the Gut Microbiota," *Nutrients* 13, no. 5 (May 2021): 1655, https://www.ncbi.nlm.nih.gov/pmc/articles/PMC8153313/.

SEAFOOD

1. Bo Zhang et al., "Fish Consumption and Coronary Heart Disease: A Meta-Analysis," *Nutrients* 12, no. 8 (July 2020): 2278, https://www.mdpi.com/2072-6643/12/8/2278.

2. "Eating Fish Associated with Significant Health Benefits: Pooled Analysis," *Cardiovascular Journal of Africa* 32, no. 4 (July–August 2021): 227–31, https://www.ncbi.nlm.nih.gov/pmc/articles/PMC8756069/.

Index

About the Author

Noom is a consumer-first digital health platform that empowers its users to achieve holistic health outcomes through behavior change and the latest in modern medicine. Founded in 2008, Noom's mission is to help people everywhere lead healthier lives. Fueled by a powerful combination of technology, psychology, and human coaching, Noom is backed by more than a decade of user research and product development. Today, Noom's platform includes four core programs: Noom Weight for weight management; Noom Med, an enhancement to Noom Weight for obesity care; Noom Mood for stress management; and Noom DPP for diabetes prevention. Headquartered in New York City, Noom has been named one of *Inc.*'s Best Places to Work and *Fortune*'s Best Workplaces in Technology. Learn more by visiting Noom.com.

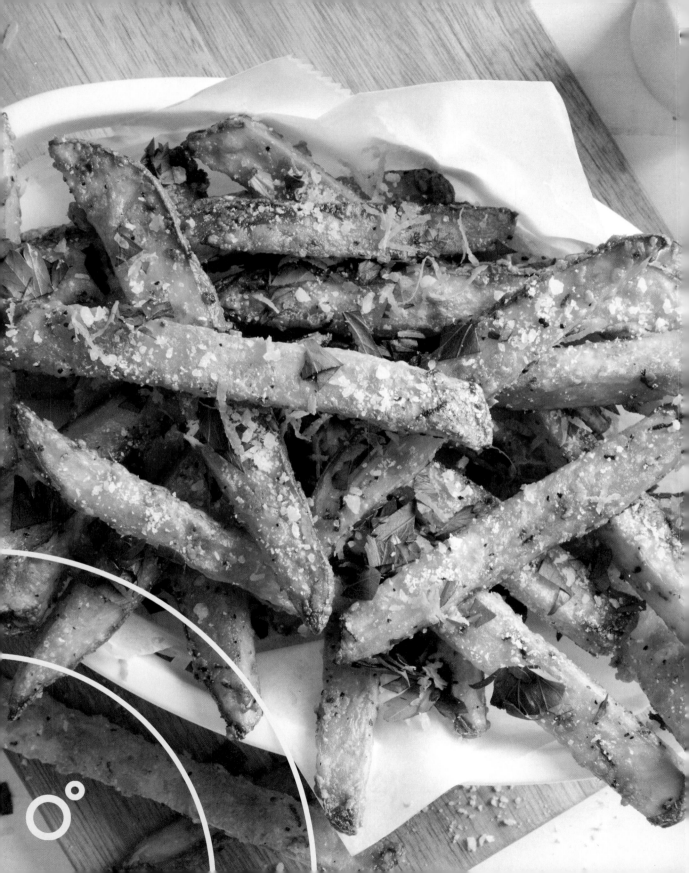